YOUR HEART

Are you taking care of it?

Holly Fourchalk, PhD., DNM®, RHT, HT

CHOICES UNLIMITED
FOR
HEALTH AND WELLNESS

This book includes neither an exhaustive nor exclusive list of alternative options for working with the health of your heart.

Rather, it provides an overview of theories, foods, herbs and modalities with which the patient or practitioner may work.

My company is called Choices Unlimited for Health and Wellness for a reason. There are lots of choices to choose from with regard to maximizing your health. We can only make good, effective choices when we have a working knowledge of what those choices may be.

If a given modality or protocol resonates for you, research it further. Explore your options within the profile. Your mind is a very powerful tool – make it work for you. Regardless of what you choose to do, make the placebo effect – or the power of the mind – be a part of your healing journey.

Here's to your journey into health.

DISCLAIMER

Every effort has been made by the author to ensure that the information in this book is as accurate as possible. However, it is by no means a complete or exhaustive examination of all information.

The author knows what worked for her and what has worked for others but no two people are the same and so the author cannot and does not render judgment or advice regarding a particular individual.

Further, because our bodies are unique any two individuals may experience different results from the same therapy.

The author believes in both prevention and the superiority of a natural non-invasive approach over drugs and surgery.

The information collected within comes from a variety of researchers and sources from around the world. This information has been accumulated in the Western healing arts over the past thirty years.

Research has shown that one of the top three leading causes of death in North America occurs because of the physician/pharmaceutical component of the scenario.

Perhaps the real leading cause of death and disability is a result of the lack of awareness of natural therapies. These therapies are well known to prevent and treat many common degenerative, inflammatory and oxidative diseases.

The author loves to research and loves to teach. This book is another attempt to increase awareness about health and the many options we have to bring the body back into a healthy balance.

Ever-increasing numbers of people are aware of healing foods and herbs, supplements and modalities but there are still far too many who are not. The fact that our physicians are part of this latter group makes healing even more challenging yet we are now seeing more and more laboratories around the world and more universities in and outside of the U.S. studying herbs, nutrition and various healing modalities with phenomenal success.

The unfortunate fact is, those who can profit from sickness and disease promote ignorance and the results are devastating.

It is not the intent of the author that anyone should choose to read this book and make decisions regarding their health or medical care based on ideas contained in this book.

It is the responsibility of the individual to find a health care practitioner to work with to achieve optimal health.

The author and publisher are not responsible for any adverse effects or consequences resulting from the use of any of the suggestions or information contained in the book but offer this material as information that the public has a right to hear and utilize at its own discretion.

To my Parents

For all their support and encouragement
My Dad for his ever-listening ear
My mother for her open mind

CONTENTS

ONE

What about your heart?

This book is going to use the same format as my previous books. It will include:

- An introduction to the heart
- An understanding of how the heart functions
- What can go wrong with the cardiovascular system
- What can cause those problems
- What we can do to solve the problems

The heart has a unique place in most cultures. It is really the only organ that is associated with an emotion in western society. We usually associate the emotion love with the heart. Books are written about this heart love. We have holidays surrounding the heart, i.e. Valentine's Day. Just think for a moment…what emotion do you associate with the kidney, the pancreas, or the spleen?

Yet in **Traditional Chinese Medicine** (TCM) each organ system/meridian is associated with a different emotion (Note: There is not a direct association between the TCM meridian and the organ.)

- *Liver*: Anger — indigestion, diarrhea, depression
- *Heart*: Joy — too much or stress, plus palpitations, anxiety, insomnia

1

- *Lungs*: Sadness—fatigue, shortness of breath, depression

- *Spleen*: Worry—digestive issues, chronic fatigue

- *Kidneys*: Fear—bladder issues

- *Adrenals*: Fight/flight—kidneys/heart

Or in **Ayurvedic medicine** (East Indian Medicine – the oldest known medicine to mankind) we have three basic styles of operating:

- *Vata* style of operating: Worry, fear, anxiety, insecurity

- *Pitta* style of operating: Anger, hatred, envy, jealousy, competitiveness, aggression, judgment, criticism

- *Kapha* style of operating: Attachment, greed

And then we have:

- *Liver*—anger

- *Gallbladder*—hate

- *Lung*—grief, sadness

- *Kidneys*—fear

- *Colon*—anxiety

In conventional medicine, we are taught that the brain was responsible for these emotional functions, in particular, the limbic system. However, in recent years we have discovered that there are over 90 known neuropeptides (proteins) that are not just secreted by the brain but also secreted by the cells in the body.

These protein molecules serve as mediators of mental activity and can change action and physiology. Once again, "modern medicine" is beginning to understand what the different ancient healing modalities knew thousands of years ago.

Likewise, we associate the brain with thoughts and cognitive functions but not with other organs. Yet, if the liver is not functioning, we can have cognitive impairment. If the gut is not working we can cognitive impairment. If the adrenals are not working we can have cognitive impairment, too, and so on.

In TCM we have:

- *Wood*: Liver/gallbladder — clear vision and goals, planning and decision-making

- *Fire:* Heart/small intestine — self-expression, consciousness, memories, concern for self and others, leadership

- *Earth:* Stomach/spleen — contentment, mediation, self-discipline

- *Metal*: Lung/Colon — inspiration, meaning, confidence, achievers

- *Water*: Kidney/Bladder — will power, wisdom, actualization, determination

Scientific evidence continues to understand more and more as it unravels the complexity of the human system. But what is even more exciting is how, in so many ways, science continues to validate the theories of old ways.

Even current theories are still in conflict over whether the brain contains or reflects the mind. Now they are starting to look at whether what we thought belonged to the brain really does and asking if it is in different parts of the body, or perhaps in energy fields.

We are obviously not just a combination of Newtonian chemicals that operate in a mechanistic manner but a wonderfully interactive, inter-dynamic, and intercon-nected much more than western medicine believed us to be.

Obviously, in this book, we are going to concentrate on the heart. So let's look at what western culture attributes to the heart.

We have all kinds of saying and quotes regarding the heart:

Attraction:

- Big-hearted

- Heart throb

- Sweetheart

Philosophy:

- Heart of the matter

- Home is where the heart is

- "One of the hardest things in life is having words in your heart that you can't utter." James Earl

- "A fool with a heart and no sense is just as unhappy as a fool with sense and no heart." Fyodor Dostoyevsky, The Idiot

- "One love, one heart, one destiny." Bob Marley

- "The heart has its reasons which reason knows not." Blaise Pascal

4

- "When the heart speaks, the mind finds it indecent to object." Milan Kundera

Emotion:

- Broken heart
- Heartbroken
- Heart-sick
- Heart sore
- Heart-warming
- Heavy-hearted
- "If only my heart were stone." Cormac McCarthy, The Road
- "Life will not break your heart. It'll crush it." Henry Rollins

Other emotions:

- Chicken-hearted
- Faint-hearted
- Happy-hearted
- Lighthearted

Personality:

- Big-hearted
- Bold hearted
- Hard-hearted
- Heartless
- Heart of gold

- Lion-hearted
- Open-hearted
- Soft-hearted
- Wild-hearted

Biblical:

- "Where your treasure is, there will your heart be also." Holy Bible

Health issues:

- Heart attack
- Heartburn

We even use the St. Valentine's icon of the heart to mean we "love" something. This apparently began in 1977 with:

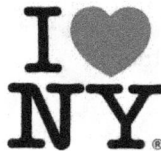

I ♥ NY

The usage of the symbol goes back to the Coat of Arms of Denmark in 12th century and the first depiction of the shape as a heart metaphor began in the 13th and 14th century according to Wikipedia.[2]

Why is the heart so important that we have so many sayings and quotes, icons, and images about this organ? Well, just as we have associated the brain with cognitive processes, we have attributed the heart with emotion. In particular, we usually associate the heart with loving emotions. But does emotion reside in the heart?

In Traditional Chinese Medicine, each organ system is associated with different emotions. For instance, the liver is associated with anger, and the lungs with sadness.

Think of when you "feel" or "experience" an emotion. Is it in the heart? Now if the emotion is intense, you may feel the heart beat faster but the same is as true of love and it is of anger. Typically, when we "feel" an emotion, we feel it with our whole body, like when you get goose bumps, or when someone says something that "hits a nerve". The goose bumps spread throughout your body just as the emotion spreads throughout your body.

In fact, we may even go so far as to say we "feel" emotion with our gut more than anything. We may "feel" those "warm fuzzies" in our tummies but we don't feel them in our hearts. So where did this association between love and the heart come from?

When we pull apart the different definitions and/or experiences of love, the question becomes even more complex. Most languages have a number of different words identifying different types of love. For instance, there are the five types of love in Greek: *Agape,* meaning an ideal type of pure love rather than physical attraction; *Eros,* meaning passionate, sensual desire and longing; *Philia,* meaning loyalty, virtue, equality and familiarity; *Storge,* meaning a natural affection; and *Xenia,* meaning hospitality.

In Buddhism, we have *Kama* meaning sensuous love and *Karuna* meaning compassion.

7

English appears to be the most lacking it its capacity to differentiate different types of love. However, when discussing a romanticized or sexualized love we do have: Infatuation, being in love, and loving. But this does not provide us with a differentiation when saying "I love ice cream" (a food) or, "I love my dog" (a pet) or, "I love my car" (something material) or, "I love philosophy" (something abstract) or, "I love God" (religious or spiritual).

According to Wikipedia again:

"Love refers to a variety of different feelings, states, and attitudes that ranges from interpersonal affection ("I love my mother") to pleasure ("I loved that meal"). It can refer to an emotion of a strong attraction and personal attachment. It can also be a virtue representing human kinds, compassion and affection – "the unselfish loyal and benevolent concern for the good of another". It may also describe compassionate and affectionate actions towards other humans, one's self or animals". http://en.wikipedia.org/wiki/Love

If there is a physiological arousal we may experience an adrenaline rush causing a shortness of breath and/or rapid heartbeat but that would be more indicative of infatuation as opposed to being "in love" which comes with more compassion, affection, deeper understanding, and connection than infatuation.

Now from a psychological perspective, we might want to explore the differences between:

- Being infatuated

- Being in love

8

- Loving

- Caring

Unfortunately, that goes beyond the scope of this book, and may take volumes.

The flip side of the coin is when there is a breakup of this romanticized/sexualized experience of love. We may feel heartache. (Does your heart actually ache?) We may experience physiological variables such as the heart pounding but we may also experience tears, which is a central nervous system reaction, a clenched gut, nausea, and more.

The Japanese have even identified a new syndrome called the "broken heart syndrome" or takotsubo and apparently represents about 2% of what appears to be typical heart attacks? It is an adrenaline stress-induced cardiomyopathy caused by major stress such as the death of a loved one. But that means there is an interconnection between the brain, the adrenals, and the heart. It certainly takes more than the typical allopathic reductionist thinking to understand that connection.

We even have professional books about how to heal a broken heart. Cans the heart actually break?

Recent science concerning the "atlas of human emotions" doesn't agree with this. Researchers in Finland have studied fourteen human emotions with over 700 subjects who were asked to paint two representations, on a computer, of the emotional experience—one as it increased and the other as it decreased. When the data was compiled they were able to come up with images of fourteen different emotions and how they were experienced over the body.[1]

So where does the connection between love and the heart come in? Why have we attributed it to the heart?

Ayurvedic or East Indian medicine/philosophy may have the answer. While these modalities identify over 109 chakras/energy wheels throughout the body, there are seven major ones that occur up the spine. They attribute the "Heart Chakra" to compassion, healing, romantic love, and unconditional love.

So perhaps this association has nothing to do with the physiology of the heart but rather an association between the chakra that falls at the heart level and the emotions or issues associated with this particular chakra.

Again, the point is, there is a lot of interaction going on here and nothing in the body or mind happens in isolation.

Older medicinal practices, whether they be identified as alternative, traditional medicines, eastern, Ayurvedic, or Traditional Chinese Medicine, all acknowledged the incredible connections between different organs and systems in the body. They also had a much better understanding of the connection between the mind, emotions, and the body than we do today in the western world.

Conventional medicine, on the other hand, is terrifically reductionist and therefore, incredibly limited.

TWO

What is the cardio system?

- Primary – heart, lungs, arteries, veins
- Secondary – brain, liver, kidneys, bones

The term "cardio" originates from the Greek word "*kardia*" which means, "heart".

Now let's focus on the physical organ called the heart and the cardio system of which it is a part.

The heart is one of the few organs of which we can have a direct experience. When it beats hard or irregularly we are directly aware of it. If the kidneys, or the liver, or the pancreas function faster or slow down most of us have no perception of it.

The cardio system is a very inter-dependent system. As with all other systems and organs in the body, nothing operates in isolation but rather in a beautiful inter-dependent synchrony of systems.

The cardio system has primary and secondary systems and organs that are part of it. So let's take a quick look and understand what each component contributes to the cardio system.

The Primary Cardio system includes:

- Heart:
  - o Takes in the de-oxygenated blood from the veins
  - o Pumps the de-oxygenated blood into the lungs

- o Pumps out the oxygenated blood from the lungs
- o Pumps out the oxygenated blood into the arteries
- Lungs
  - o Takes out the CO2 from the blood
  - o Exchanges the CO2 for oxygen
- Vascular system
  - o Consists of the arteries, veins and blood
- Arteries/vascular system
  - o Carries the oxygenated blood from the heart throughout the body
  - o Uses smooth muscles that expand and contract to help move the blood
- Veins/vascular system
  - o Carries the de-oxygenated blood back to the heart
  - o Uses valves that open and close to help move the blood
- Blood/vascular system
  - o Red blood cells carry oxygen and C02
  - o White blood cells are part of the immune system
  - o Protein transport mechanisms
  - o Coagulators

The Secondary Cardio system includes:

- Kidneys

- o Cleanse the blood that travels in the vascular system thus creating the urine (thus also regulating the pH; regulation of blood pressure)

- Liver

  - o The liver's over 500 functions includes:

- Synthesizing blood proteins, i.e. albumin
- Regulation of blood sugars
- Regulating cholesterols
- Synthesizing blood coagulators
- Breaking down old red blood cells
- Cleans the blood of toxins and prepares them for elimination through either the stool or urine
- Produces hormones, i.e. antitensinogen (involved in regulating blood pressure)

- Spleen

  - o Another blood filtering organ

  - o Also breaks down old red blood cells

  - o Synthesizes antibodies for the lymph system that protect the heart

  - o Provides a reservoir for macrophages (an immune protecting compound)

- Bones

  - o Produce blood cells

  - o Can store toxic metals to protect the heart and other organs

  - o Regulates phosphate (which acts on the kidneys)

o Stores minerals like calcium and phosphorous that impact on the heart

o Secrete a hormone called osteocalcin that is involved in the regulation of blood sugar and fat deposition

That's a pretty interactive system but is only a basic understanding of what the separate organ systems do. It's a lot more complicated than that.

Let's look at just the heart:

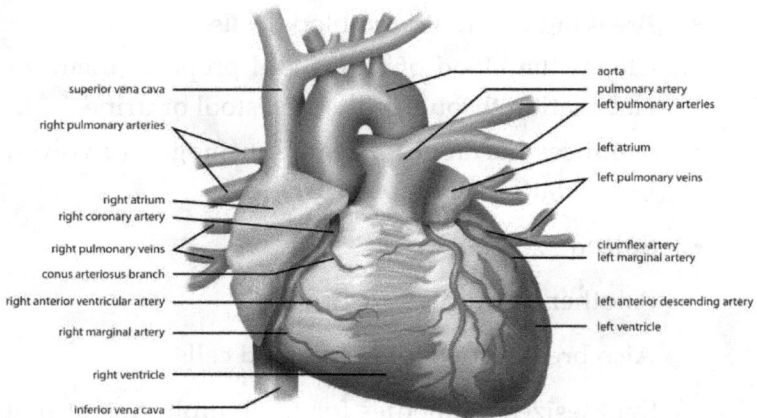

(From Wikipedia.org/wiki/heart)

Isn't it interesting that the organ looks nothing like the heart icon we use for Valentine's Day. The heart is actually a hollow muscular organ that contracts and expands in order to pump blood through four compartments:

1. From the Vena cava (vein) into the right atrium

2. From the right atrium into the right ventricle

3. From the right ventricle into the lung

4. From the lung into the left atrium

5. From the left atrium into the left ventricle

6. From the left ventricle into the aorta (artery)

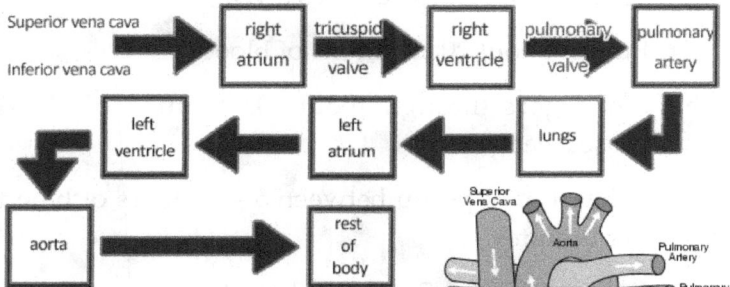

Circulation of Blood Through the Heart:

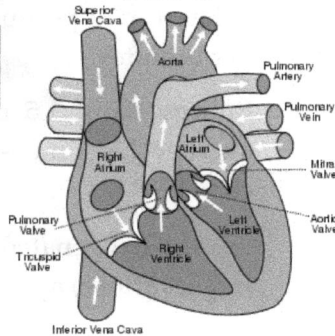

From http://en.wikipedia.org/wiki/Heart

The manner in which this is done incorporates:

1. Valves (Four of them: tricuspid, pulmonary, mitral, aorta)

2. Electrical pulse (Sinoatrial SA node)

The heart pumps about seventy-two beats per minute (2.5 million times during an average 66 lifespan) to pump 4.7 – 5.7 litres of blood per minute! Wow!

This is a good time to look at some heart facts.

• Heart begins to pump at 4 weeks after conception and continues until death

- Only stops beating when you have a hiccup
- Beats about 72 beats per minute
- Beats about 100,000 times per day
- Beats about 3,600,000 times a year
- Pumps about 2000 gallons of blood
- Blood goes through about 60,000 miles of blood vessels each day
- A heart may pump between 5 – 30 liters of blood per minutes
- Pumps about 1.5 million barrels of blood in an average life time – enough to fill 200 train tank cars
- Pumps oxygenated blood through the aorta (the largest artery) at about 1 mph or 1.6 km per hour
- 5% of the blood actually supplies the heart: 15-20% goes to the brain and central nervous system; 22% goes to the kidneys
- Weighs about 11 ounces
- The heart creates enough energy, each day, to drive a truck about 20 miles
- The heart can continue to pump outside of the body because it has its own electrical pump – as long as it has enough oxygen
- The heart pumps blood to about 100 trillion cells
- Prolonged lack of sleep can cause irregular jumping heartbeats

- A woman's heart beats faster than a man's (78 to 70)

- When the body is at rest, it takes the blood about:

  o 6 seconds to go from the heart to the lungs and back

  o 8 seconds to go to the brain and back

  o 16 seconds to go the toes and back

- Cocaine can alter the electrical current of the heart causing a heart attack or stroke[1]

This makes for great trivia for the cocktail party but what is important here is that your heart/cardiovascular system needs nutrients to achieve all that.

1. Every cell in the body has a multitude of organs called organelles. One of the organelles is called the mitochondria. This organelle is responsible for producing all the fuel for each given cell so the cell can:

   - Absorb nutrients through the cell membrane
   - Create the enzymes necessary to metabolize nutrients
   - Create the transport mechanisms to move the nutrients
   - Metabolize and eliminate or resolve the toxins produced as by-products of normal functioning or what has been absorbed into the cell
   - And a 100 other functions

2. The number of mitochondria in a given cell correlates with the amount of fuel/ATP the cell requires in order to function.

3. Any given heart cell will have between 1000 – 2500 mitochondria in order to produce enough energy/fuel/ATP to keep functioning 24/7.

So, what nutrients do the heart cells need to:

4. Do all of its basic functioning as a normal cell?

5. Create, support and protect the mitochondria?

6. Allow the mitochondria to produce the ATP?

Let's read on and find out what kinds of cardiovascular issues can occur.

THREE

What kinds of cardiovascular issues can occur?

A variety of different of issues can affect our cardiovascular systems. However, while they all have the heart in common, there are differences. Let's look at some of them.

1. **Angina:**
   - *Symptoms:*
     - Causes pain
     - Tightness in the chest area
   - *Causes:*
     - Arteries are not supplying the blood
     - Arteries are narrow
     - Arteries are stiff

2. **Congenital Heart Disease** (heart abnormalities present since birth; may involve any component of the cardiovascular system))
   - *Symptoms:*
     - Bluish skin
     - Fatigue
     - Rapid heartbeat
     - Shortness of breath
     - Swelling in the abdomen

- Swelling around the eyes
  - *Causes:*
    - Viral infections
    - Medications
    - Chemicals
    - Alcohol
    - Unknown causes

3. **Congestive heart failure (the heart is losing its ability to pump)**
   - *Symptoms:*
     - Dizziness
     - Edema (swelling in feet, ankles, legs
     - Eventual disability
     - Fatigue
     - Shortness of breath
     - Weight gain
   - *Causes:*
     - Damage caused by a heart attack
     - High blood pressure
     - Diabetes
     - Coronary artery disease
     - Cancer treatments
     - Kidneys issues (not filtering the blood)
     - Toxicity (heavy metal toxins)

4. **Coronary microvascular disease (MVD)** or **microangiopathy** is a small vessel disease that damages the lining of the arteries and causes narrowing.

  o *Symptoms:*
  - Chest pain (angina)
  - Fatigue
  - Shortness of breath

  o *Causes:*
  - Diabetes
    - Diabetic retinopathy
    - Diabetic nephropathy
  - AGEs (advanced glycation endproducts)

5. **Cyanotic heart disease (results in low blood oxygen)**

  o *Symptoms:*
  - Fainting
  - Hyperventilation
  - Puffy eyes or face
  - Skin turns a blush color

  o *Causes:*
  - Valve defects
  - Hypoplastic left heart syndrome
  - Infections/medications during pregnancy

6. **Hypertensive heart disease (high blood pressure)**

- *Causes:*

  - Angina

  - Arrhythmias

  - Coronary artery disease

  - Heart attacks

  - Heart failure

- **Types:**

- **Ischemic heart disease** (reduced blood supply)

  - Traditionally this meant cholesterol issues – this will be further discussed in Chapter 5

  - Anything that narrows the arteries

  - Anything that prevents the arteries from expanding / contracting

- **Inflammatory heart disease**

  - *Symptoms:*

  - Angina

  - Fatigue

  - Shortness of breath

  - Swelling in the feet/ankles

  - *Caused by:*

    - Traditionally this meant inflammation of the heart muscles or surrounding tissues.

- o **Organic Heart Disease**
  - ▪ *Causes:*
    - ▪ Deformity
    - ▪ Inflammation
- o **Pulmonary heart disease**
  - ▪ *Causes:*
    - ▪ Blood flow from heart to lung is slow or blocked
    - ▪ Increases blood pressure to the lungs
    - ▪ Congestive heart failure
    - ▪ Lung disease affects the heart[1]

We know the vascular system that takes the blood from the heart and back to the heart can also cause problems.

In general, a vascular issue is any that affects the effectiveness of the circulatory system and usually as a result, puts more strain on the heart.

"Smooth muscles" occur in the lining of the arteries and are responsible for making the arteries expand or "vasodilate". This movement of expanding and contracting pushes the oxygenated blood through the body.

Veins, on the other hand, have valves that push the de-oxygenated blood back to the heart.

So here are some of the common vascular issues:

- • **Peripheral Artery disease**
  - o *Symptoms:*

23

- Chest pain (angina)
- Heart attack
- If in the carotid artery that supplies the brain:
- Transient ischemic attack (TIAs)
- If in the legs
- Legs cramps/pain
- Changes in skin color
- Sores/ulceration
- Tired legs
- Gangrene/loss of a leg
- If in the renal (kidneys) arteries:
- Hypertension
- Heart failure
- Abnormal kidney function
  - *Causes:*
    - Traditionally it was thought to be caused by atherosclerosis — plaque along the inner lining of the arteries.
    - The cholesterol myth will be further explored in Chapter 5.
- **Aneurysm: (localized blood filled bulge in the wall of the blood vessel)**
  - *Symptoms — if in the brain:*
    - Double vision

- Fatigue

- Loss of balance

- Loss of perception

- Neck pain and/or stiffness

- Pain above/behind the eyes

- Speech issues

o *Symptoms* — *if in the kidneys:*

- Flank pain/tenderness (between ribs and hips)

- Red blood cells in the urine

- Hypertension

- Signs of hypovolemic shock

o *Symptoms* — *if in the abdomen:*

- Central back pain

- Edema (swelling in the ankles/ feet)

- Vomiting

o *Cause:*

- An abnormal bulge in the wall of a blood vessel. These usually occur in the aorta vessel – either in the thoracic aorta or the abdominal aorta.

- **Renal/Kidney artery disease**

o *Cause:*

- Traditionally thought to be caused by atherosclerosis

- Will be further explored in Chapter xx
- Sometimes can be caused by congenital defect
- Blood clots in the veins
  - *Causes:*
    - Congestive heart failure
    - Damage to veins (injury or infection)
    - Damage to valves in veins
    - Hormones (birth control or estrogens)
    - Long periods of bed rest or immobility
    - Pregnancy
    - Surgery[2]

Note how many symptoms are similar across different diagnoses. So what do we need to conclude?

1. Whenever an issue causes more pressure to be put on the heart — there is a risk.

2. Whenever oxygen doesn't get to a given location, especially the brain that uses about 20% of the body's oxygen — there is a problem.

But we are always hearing about cholesterol and how many people are taking anti-cholesterol or statin drugs. So, let's take a look at cholesterol.

FOUR

What can cause nutrient deficiency?

A wide number of compounds and practices in today's world can cause nutritional deficiency. Let's go over some of the most prevalent ones.

Nutrient deficiency:

Nutrient deficiency can be the result of a poor diet. It can be caused by the lack of nutritionally rich foods that have been grown in depleted soils. In the old days, farmers used a five- or seven-year crop rotation cycle on their land. This ensured that there were always different crops available for sell *and* that the soil had a chance to recover its nutrient value.

In today's world, we no longer have the crop rotations and the soils are appallingly depleted of important minerals and phytonutrients. Instead, farmers often must attempt to replenish the soil using harsh chemicals, plus adding pesticides, herbicides, and insecticides. While in the air, persistent organic pollutants, (POP) are travelling around the world and getting absorbed into plants along the way.

If this were not bad enough, we now have all the GMO seeds (genetically modified organisms) that have already been shown to cause all kinds of health issues.

A common example that is used to demonstrate this modern problem is a serving of broccoli. The nutrient value of one serving of broccoli taken from 50 years ago is equivalent to between 18-22 servings today (depending on the soil in which it was grown).

That is a major difference in nutrient value, wouldn't you say?

In addition to the poor soils in which our foods are grown, we have the following issues that deplete our nutrient.

Pasteurization: Most of us associate pasteurization with milk or dairy products but in fact, different forms of pasteurization are utilized on fruit and vegetables and meats. Pasteurization involves heating foods to eliminate dangerous bacteria. But in addition, pasteurization can also destroy:

- Valuable enzymes (that help us digest milk)
- Vitamins: A, C, B6, B12
- Phytonutrients, in particular phenols (anti-oxidants)
- Milk proteins
- Valuable bacteria[1,2]

Microwaving

Whether microwaves are detrimental to food nutrients appears to be rather controversial. Some claim that the damage is minimal *or* that microwaving results in the same amount of nutritional loss as steaming or stir-frying.

Some claim if the food is microwaved at a lower setting that there is as much loss or retention of nutrients as conventional ovens.

However, the majority of studies show a loss of nutrients. For instance, anti-oxidants, which are known to be sensitive to heat to begin with, appear to have the highest risk factor, i.e. up to 97% loss. Whereas steamed broccoli lost 11% of the anti-oxidants. [3]

One of the most commonly known impacts is on the proteins through a process called "protein unfolding". Microwaves are known to cause a "significant higher degree" of this protein unfolding than conventional heat.[4]

Then we have the anti-bodies. Those found in mother's milk are altered and actually make a more suitable environment for pathogenic bacteria. [5]

What about vitamins? Research has shown that microwaves turn Vitamin B12 into an inert or dead form.[6]

How about other phytonutrients? Let's look at garlic. The research shows that the microwaves inactivate one of the "active ingredients" allinase, which fights against cancer.[7]

Conclusion: While various studies suggest the microwave does not have a negative impact, when we look at individual nutrients, the studies usually indicate that there is indeed a negative impact.

Processing

First off, let's clarify what we mean by processing. After all, just pulling grapes from a tree, blending a juice, or grinding beef could be considered processing. However, there is a difference between mechanical processing and chemical processing.

In addition, there is a difference between types of chemical processing that is beneficial and others that are detrimental. For instance, fermentation is a form of processing that is beneficial to the body. We are going to focus on the types of chemical processing that are detrimental to the body.

"Processed" foods contain various oils, sweeteners like high fructose corn syrup, starches, unhealthy fats and salts, to lengthen shelf life and improve tastes. Additionally, they may also contain large quantities of chemical additives, preservatives, and flavorings.

Sodium

These processed foods also tend to have high amounts of sodium. Now, sodium is found in real whole foods but in low amounts. The high amounts found in processed food, used for preservation and taste, contribute to heart problems. There are various types of sodium:

- Sodium chloride (table salt) prevents food borne pathogens; prolongs shelf life; and helps bind ingredients; enhances food colours; improves the taste and functions as a stabilizer.

  o Sounds okay until you realize that it leads to health complications like high blood pressure, strokes and weight gain.

- Monosodium glutatmate (MSG which is a neural toxin)

30

- Sodium benzoate: A food preservative that prevents bacteria and fungal growth under various acidic conditions, found in salad dressings, carbonated drinks, fruit juices, pickles, jams and various condiments as well as prescriptions and cosmetics. The degree to which it is toxic depends on a number of variables, according to the WHO (World Health Organization).

- Sodium saccharin: According to an article in PubMed, the use of saccharin has been controversial since its discovery in 1879. This particular research study claims that the impact is not genotoxic (it does not interact with the DNA to cause cancer) but rather it effects several changes including pH, sodium, protein, and silicates, in the urinary tract).

- Sodium nitrate: A preservative used in deli meats, bacon, jerky, sausage. It is believed that the chemical damages your blood vessels and contributes to hardening of the arteries. It also impacts on the utilization of sugars in the body and may contribute to diabetes.

- Sodium bicarbonate: Otherwise known as baking soda can have many benefits to the body but can also become toxic and have unwanted side effects like headaches, loss of appetite, muscles tiredness, muscles restlessness, pain or twitching, nausea or vomiting, edema, tiredness or weakness, and breathing problems.

So while the body requires small amounts of sodium, different types of sodium have different affects on the body. Typically the kind found in processed foods are the types that are detrimental.

Fats

Fats and sugars have both taken a beating in the last few decades. Ultimately, we have to recognize that not all fats, just like not all sugars, are the same. Our bodies require various types of fats and sugars for a wide variety of reasons. But we need the good healthy ones.

The "bad fats" (cheap fats, vegetable oils, hydrogenated or trans fats, etc.) cause a lot of problems. They are difficult to metabolize, they can "clog" up the system, and they are easily oxidized. Furthermore, although we do require Omega 6 fats, we have way too much of these in the body in relation to the Omega 3s. Our diets used to have much higher levels of Omega 3s (anti-inflammatories) and therefore the body evolved or was created to take Omega 6s (pro-inflammatory) preference over Omega 3s.

Now our bodies require both the Omega 3s and the Omega 6s. But the problem today is that there are hardly any Omega 3s in our diet and we are still designed to take Omega 6s over the Omega 3s. Consequently, we have a lot more Omega 6s in the body and a deficiency in the Omega 3s. This causes all kinds of complications such as excess and chronic inflammation.

Sugars and AGEs

"Processed" foods are also usually high in sugars like high fructose corn syrup. We already know that as a society we consume way too much sugar. Further, these sugars are "empty calories" meaning non-nutritional. Further, when these sugars are heated in conjunctions with fats and/or lipids, they create advanced glycation end products or AGEs, which are extremely harmful to cells. The AGEs are even more harmful than free radicals. They attach to cells and cause cellular dysfunction and death. This is not only particularly harmful in the blood vessels but also dangerous in a number of tissues.

These sugars and AGEs are found in everything from processed foods, baking, junk food, processed foods, and all of the sugar-sweetened drinks. People then make matters even worse by putting in more sugar into their coffee and tea.

These sugars cause problems to our already overwhelmed liver, adrenals, and pancreas. They drain our body of our hormones such as cortisol and insulin, which are utilized to regulate the blood glucose levels.

These sugars are associated with some major diseases and disorders, such as heart disease, diabetes, cancer, and obesity.

Artificial ingredients

Have you ever looked at the labels on foods? Do you understand all of the terms on the label? Chances are you don't. Even foods acclaimed to be healthy have a list of artificial chemicals on the packaging. There are pages of synthetic chemicals lists that are allowed to hide behind the umbrella label of "artificial flavors". They are identified as "safe" by the same regulatory bodies that claim that sugars and vegetable oils are safe.

The challenge with these ingredients is that our bodies were not created or designed to metabolize, absorb, or utilize these chemicals. We do not have enzymes to break them down or reconfigure them into effective compounds, nor the receptors to absorb them effectively. Consequently, they become toxic to the body.

The body has to find ways to eliminate them but they overwhelm the system. They may feed pathogens we don't want in our bodies. They may compete for receptors we want for good healthy nutrients; they may deplete various compounds as the body struggles to eliminate them. All in all, they are detrimental.

Refined carbohydrates

Another problem with processed foods is the high amounts of refined carbohydrates. Complex carbohydrates are good for us but simple refined carbohydrates are dangerous. They cause spiking of blood sugars in the liver along with lack of fibres to regulate them.

Again, we face challenges when reading food labels. For instance, if the label says whole grains, they are often pulverized into such fine flours that they end up being just as dangerous as refined flour.

Synthetic nutrients

What about foods that have been "fortified" with vitamins and other nutrients? First off, they are usually the artificial synthetic form of the nutrient not the form that you would actually find in the plant source.

Furthermore, when the nutrients are found in the real food, they are found in conjunction with all kinds of other nutrients (vitamins, minerals, fats, fibers, antioxidants, etc.) that operate synergistically to support both metabolism and absorption.

Taste buds — let's look at why they are important

Our taste buds are a benefit to us but the various processed food companies who compete for our purchasing can also utilize them. These manufacturers play with our sense of taste and texture to create foods that end up being harmful to our health but increase their sales. Triggering the taste buds may cause addictions or alter our senses.

We have six different types of taste buds: sweet, sour, salty, bitter, pungent, unami, and most recently, kokumi, which has been identified by Asian cultures.

Some claim that piquancy, the burn on the tongue that spicy eaters love, is also a taste sense. It and the sense of coolness are transmitted to the brain through the trigeminal nerve rather than the classical nerves identified for taste. The receptors are different from the typical taste receptors and are called TPRM1 and TPRM8. They also have an impact on taste.

Another taste that is controversial is the taste of metals or the metallic taste. It is currently believed that the perception of these metallic tastes comes through another process, i.e. electrical conductivity but again, it is a sense that is utilized.

What about fatty foods? Is that a perception of texture or a taste perception? Apparently we have "varying taste thresholds for fatty acids, the long chains that along with glycerol comprise fats, or lipids". [8]

What about carbon dioxide? That is the chemical that is dissolved in liquids to create the bubbly sensation in soda drinks, beer, champagne, etc. Historically, it was believed that the tingling sensation was stimulating the trigeminal nerve and thus it wasn't really a taste bud but this idea is being challenged, too. Regardless of what it is doing or how it is being perceived, it is certainly a mechanism that the various beverage companies utilize to provoke us to buy their products.

Ultimately, the more man "messes" with our food and nutrition, the more they become detrimental to our bodies. It doesn't matter whether it is through pasteurization, microwaving, or chemical processing, these altered "foods" that we put into our bodies, do the following:

- Destroy good nutrients
- Use up our good nutrients for processing, or eliminating them
- Compete with healthy nutrients for transport mechanisms
- Cause problems with excess:
  - Free radicals
  - AGEs
  - Inflammation
- Provide our bodies with calories but without nutrients

The more processing, the fewer good whole nutrients we get. We end up with less and less nutrient value and more and more detrimental value. These detrimental effects can have a huge negative impact on our whole cardiovascular system. On top of the incredible nutrient deficiency, we have to add all the toxicity.

Toxicity

Toxicity can come into the body in a variety of ways. First, it has been purported that over 80,000 toxic chemicals have been introduced since the onset of the Industrial Revolution. The Environmental Protection Agency (EPA) claims that hundreds more are introduced each year. That's a lot of toxins, wouldn't you agree? Over 77,000 of them are in active production in North America. Many of these have been banned in other countries. Toxins can have a variety of different damages affects in our bodies. For instance:

1. Toxins can attach to cells and prevent them from functioning properly and/or kill them.

2. Toxins can interfere with the functioning of other compounds.

3. Toxins can attach to the lining of the blood vessels and cause inflammation.

4. Toxins can interfere with any muscle's capacity to expand and contract.

5. Toxins can interfere with the immune system's functioning and ability to protect us against pathogens.

6. Toxins can interfere with hormone production and regulation.

7. Toxins can create developmental abnormalities.

8. Toxins can neural damage.

9. Toxins can cause nerve damage.

10. Toxins provoke various dysfunctions in cells, organs, tissues and systems.

11. Toxins can deplete our bodies of the nutrients that our bodies require.

What is perhaps even scarier are the claims that over 60% of these are found in our homes.

1. Food toxicity:

1. PCBs:

- Herbicides: Recent studies show that herbicides, like *Roundup,* that are used on agricultural grain farms can cause DNA damage, endocrine disruption, and cell death. When inert chemicals/ingredients are mixed with glyphosate, they are able to cross cell membrane in plants and humans. Remember, they are designed to kill.[9]

- Pesticides: Pesticide residues are detectable in 50-95% of food consumed in the US. [10]

- Insecticides: Are not readily bioavailable and affect the nervous system as stimulants/convulsants, 2 organochlorine (lindane and methoxychlor) and still have limited use. [11]

2. Dioxins: 90% of our exposure to dioxins is found in the food chain (meat, dairy, fish, and shellfish) and can cause cancer, developmental problems, and interfere with hormones and the immune system.[12]

   - Dioxins, PCBs, organchlorine, and mercury are all found in farm raised salmon. [13]

3. POPs: Persistent organic pollutants, a.k.a. PB (Persistant Bioaccumulative) a.k.a. TOMPs (toxic organic micro pollutants) are obviously persistent and travel the globe. They can be transported by wind, water, species, and mother's milk. The dirty dozen consists of: aldrin, chlordane, dichloro-diphenyl trichloroethane, dieldrin, endrin, hepta-chlor, hexachlorobenzene, mirex, toxaphene, polychlorinated biphenyls/dibenzo-p-dioxins /furans. They cause: reproductive, develop-mental, behavioral, neurological, endocrine, and immunological dysfunctions. [14]

4. Plastics: Plastic wraps and bottles contain phthalates that mimic hormones and can damage the endocrine system.

5. Heavy metals: Heavy metals can come through a variety of foods and they have a compound effect. The effect is different depending on which has the highest toxicity level. [15, 16]

   i. Mercury
      - Fish – salmon, tuna
      - High Fructose corn syrup
      - Rice (when grown near industry) [17]

ii. Lead
- Drinking water
- Imported foods from China, Mexico, i.e. grown near industry
- Foods stored in ceramics, pottery, china or crystal
- Children's food and Baby foods [18,19]

iii. Arsenic
- From organic rice to baby food, rice breakfast cereals, brown/white rice (Arkansas, Louisiana, Missouri, Texas
  - Apple and grape juice [20]
  - Fruits and vegetables, grains, seafood[21]
  - Chicken [22]

iv. Aluminum
- Food additives
- Flour
- Baking powder
- Colouring agents
- Anti-caking agents [23]

6. Hormone injections:

- The US uses Bovine growth hormone (BGH) to stimulate milk production. Note: "dairy cows used to live 25 years. Now, few make it past 4 years because of the BGH they are injected with". [24]
- Chicken and meat also contain growth hormone. (What do you think they do to your body?)

But we are not only attacking our bodies and our hearts with toxicities from our foods, we also have to consider:

Environmental toxicity:

- The air we breathe: Coal gas, asbestos, silicon dioxide, lead, arsenic, mercury, PCBs, are in the very air we breathe.
- Carpets: Contain volatile organic compounds (VOCs), which typically outgases more than twelve chemicals, i.e. benzene, which is known to cause leukemia.
- Pressed wood products: Whether paneling, particleboard, or insulation, urea formaldehyde is used to hold them together and can cause cancer.
- Laser printers release ultra-fine particles that can cause serious health problems, again VOCs, which have been linked to heart and lung disease.
- Paint: Contains lead, which the US government claimed to be the greatest environmental threat to children and is particularly dangerous if the paint begins to peel away.
- Flame retardants: Polybrominated diphenyl ethers (PBDEs) are used in computer and television casings, upholstery, and mattresses.
- Air fresheners/cleaning solutions: Contain two particular toxins—ethylene-based glycol ethers and terpenes. When terpenes combine with ozone in the air it forms poisons. Air

fresheners have a variety of VOCs, i.e. nitric oxide and paradichlorobene.

- Baby bottles contain polycarbonate plastics with bisphenol-a (BPA), which acts as a hormone disruptor because of its similarity to estrogen.

Personal hygiene toxicity:

- Phthalates: Used in everything from deodorants, shampoos, hair spray, and fragrances — hormone disrupters.
- Sodium lauryl sulphate: Cleansers, shampoos, bubble bath, and toothpaste, found in 90% of personal care products.
- Lead: Found in personal care products and cosmetics linked to cancer and allergies.
- EWG (Environmental Working Group) has over 73,000 products listed with their toxic analysis. Go to: http://www.ewg.org/skindeep/site/about.php.[25]

Household cleaning toxicity:

- Whether to fight germs, streaks, stains, or odours, we use products that are hazardous to our health. 2-Butoxyethanol, coal tar dyes, MEA, DEA, TEA, phthalates, NPEs, phosphates, Quats, etc. all can cause a wide range of damages. [26]
- Pesticides kill everything from microorganisms to rodents.

Medical and Dental toxicity:

- APT (Acute pharmaceutical toxicity): The more drugs you take, the greater the compound effect, and the more dangerous they become.[27]
  - Unfortunately, studies look at the impact of just one synthetic toxic drug, not the compound effect of either combining the effect of various toxic compounds, or prescribing pharmaceutical cocktails!
- Amalgams: Dental fillings not only contain mercury but other toxic metals such as silver, tin, copper, zinc.[28]
- Vaccinations: From formaldehyde to aluminum phosphate to MSG to thimerosal, vaccinations are full of toxic ingredients.[29]

EPA (Environmental Protection Agency) has shown that 100% of the people tested have these in their bodies:

- Dioxins

- PCBs

- Dichlorobenzene

- Xylene

- Benzene (89% of the population)

- Percholoethlylene (93% of the population)

Worse than that, various studies have looked at infants and the umbilical cord, and found horrible toxicities. One study done by the EPA scanned the umbilical cords of ten infants born between August and September of 2004 in various US hospitals and the test results showed that the blood samples contained:

- 287 toxins and chemical pollutants, 200 on average per sample.
- 28 waste products, such as dioxins and furans, chemicals that come out of smoke stacks.
- 47 consumer product ingredients, such as flame-retardants from furniture and clothing, Teflon chemicals, and pesticides.
- 212 industrial chemicals and breakdown products from pesticides that have been banned for 30 years or longer.

The mere presence of a toxin doesn't automatically mean it is doing damage, but the ten Americans study findings raise concern, Cook said, because of the chemicals found:

- 134 have shown to cause cancer in lab animals or people
- 151 are associated with causing birth defects
- 154 are endocrine disruptors, they interfere with the body's hormonal system and produce adverse developmental, reproductive, neurological, and immune effects
- 186 are linked to infertility
- 130 are immune system toxins
- 158 are neurotoxins [30]

Research is only just starting to look at the compound effect of these toxins.

Whether these chemicals come through the air, through our gastrointestinal tract, or through our skin, they create toxicity in the blood.

Most of them make their way to the liver, which normally does the majority of detoxification. The liver does its best to chelate and/or detoxify these chemicals so that they body can eliminate them. However, many of them cannot be eliminated and end up migrating throughout the body.

Our fat cells are usually very cooperative and protective and hide the chemicals inside so that they don't harm the body.

The totality of all these chemicals is called the "total toxic burden" and can lead to all kinds of disorders, dysfunctions, and nutrient depletions in the body.

So, what does all of this have to do with the heart? Well, all of these chemicals take a ride in your cardiovascular system, i.e. in your blood. They can travel the entire expanse of your body and certainly travel through your heart. What kind of damage can these toxins cause? Oh dear, the list is so long it would take volumes to explore all of them. Let's look at some basic issues.

Symptoms of heavy metal poisoning:

- Alcohol intolerance
- Allergies: environmental
- Allergies: food
- Anxious/irritable
- Brain fog
- Coated tongue

45

- Cold hands/feet
- Dark circles under eyes
- Depression
- Digestive issues
- Extreme fatigue
- Frequent colds/flu
- Headaches
- High levels of toxic metals in blood/urine or tissues
- Insomnia
- Intolerance: meds/vitamins
- Loss of memory/forgetfulness
- Low body temperature
- Metallic taste in mouth
- Muscle and joint pain
- Muscle tics and twitches
- Muscle tremors
- Night sweats
- Parasites
- Prone to mood swings
- Prone to rashes
- Sensitive teeth
- Sensitive to odours
- Skin issues
- Small black spots on your gums
- Sore or receding gums
- Tingling in the extremities
- Unexplained chronic pain
- Unsteady gait

- Vitamin/mineral deficiencies
- Weight gain[31]

Medications:

We can look at medications in two different ways. One way is how heart medications can cause further heart and other problems. Or, we can look at medications in general that cause heart problems.

The following are lists of symptoms due to pharmaceutical toxicity as a result of various heart medications:

Common symptoms:

- Mental disorientation
- Dizziness
- Blurred vision
- Memory loss
- Fainting
- Falls

Cardiac glycosides:

- Blurred vision
- Halos around objects
- Hives
- Rash
- Diarrhea
- Loss of appetite
- Nausea
- Stomach pain
- Vomiting

- Irregular heartbeat
- Weakness
- Confusion
- Depression
- Disorientation
- Drowsiness
- Fainting
- Hallucinations
- Headache
- Lethargy

Digitalis:

- Confusion
- Irregular pulse
- Loss of appetite
- Nausea, vomiting, diarrhea
- Palpitations
- Vision changes

Digoxin: Treat heart failure and irregular heartbeat

- Loss of appetite
- Nausea
- Vomiting
- Diarrhea
- Blurred vision
- Confusion
- Drowsiness
- Insomnia
- Nightmares

- Agitation
- Depression
- Psychosis
- Delirium
- Nightmares
- Agitation
- Convulsions

Diltiazem: Treats high blood pressure and prevent angina

- Fainting
- Swelling ankles/feet
- Slow/irregular/pounding/fast heartbeat
- Shortness of breath
- Unusual tiredness
- Unexplained/sudden weight gain
- Mental/mood changes (such as depression, agitation)
- Unusual dreams

Heparin: Treat and/or prevent blood clots

- Pain/loss of feeling in the arms/legs
- Change in color of the arms/legs
- Chest pain
- Vision changes
- Trouble breathing
- Confusion
- Weakness on one side of the body
- Slurred speech

Furosemide/Lasix: used to reduce body fluids caused by: heart failure, liver disease and kidney disease

- Muscle cramps
- Weakness
- Unusual tiredness
- Confusion
- Severe dizziness
- Fainting
- Drowsiness
- Unusual dry mouth/thirst
- Nausea
- Vomiting
- Fast/irregular heartbeat
- Unusual decrease in the amount of urine

Lipitor/atorvastatin: a statin that reduces cholesterol levels

- Blocks production of CoQ10
- Weakness
- Chest pain
- Insomnia/dizziness
- Rash
- Abdominal pain
- Nausea
- Constipation
- Diarrhea
- Urinary tract infection
- Infections, colds, flus
- Arthralgia, myalgia, back pain

- Arthritis
- Peripheral edema
- Sinusitis, pharyngitis, bronchitis, rhinitis

Metoprolol/Lopressor: Beta-blocker used for hypertension

- Dizziness/fainting
- Drowsiness
- Unusual fatigue
- Diarrhea
- Unusual dreams
- Ataxia
- Difficulty sleeping
- Depression
- Visual issues
- Mental/mood changes
- Numbness and cold in hands/feet
- Bluish coloration in fingers and toes
- Hair loss
- Trouble breathing
- Easy bruising
- Persistent sore throat
- Fever
- Yellowing of skin/eyes
- Stomach pain
- Dark urine

Nitoglycerin: Prevent chest pain with those who have coronary artery disease

- Fainting

- Rash
- Fast/irregular/pounding heartbeat
- Itching/swelling (especially of the face/tongue/throat)
- Severe dizziness
- Trouble breathing

Plavix/clopidogrel: Used to prevent heart attacks, strokes

- Bleeding conditions (such as stomach ulcers, bleeding in the brain/eye)
- Recent surgery
- Serious injury/trauma
- Liver disease
- Bleeding disease (such as hemophilia)

Nifedipine/Procardia: calcium channel blocker used for hypertension

- Headache
- Nausea
- Dizziness or lightheadedness
- Heartburn
- Flushing (feeling of warmth)
- Fast heart beats
- Muscle cramps
- Constipation
- Decreased sexual ability
- Cough

Warfarin/Coumadin: Used to treat blood clots and/or deep vein thrombosis:

- Stomach bleeding
- Heavy bleeding
- Excessive bruising
- Osteoporosis
- Warfarin necrosis (skin and tissue death)
- Purple toe syndrome (blockages breaking loose and causing embolisms in the blood vessels)
- Calcification of values/arteries [32,33]

Other categories of medications that cause heart/cardio issues when toxic:

- Anesthetics
- Anti-depressants
- Calcium channel blockers
- Cytostatics
- Immunomodulating
- Nonsteroidal anti-inflammatories (NSAIDs)
- Calcium channel blockers [34]

The conclusion from this chapter can be one of two responses:

1. Holy cow, I give up. What is the point? I might as well just eat and medicate myself to death!

2. This is terrific! Now that I know what to avoid and what I need to take.

Let's take a look at CoQ10.

FIVE

The Cholesterol myths

- So what is the cholesterol myth?

- How did it get started?

- How come we still have it?

- What is cholesterol?

- What is it used for?

- Why do we have different types?

These are all good questions and what we are going to explore in this chapter.

Note: You may wish to read the book, *The Cholesterol Myth*, by Uffe Ravnskov, written in 2000[1] for further exploration.

You will see a good overview of the whole issue here.

The study that caused a problem

A study was done in 1950 from which the conclusion was made that high levels of cholesterol caused atherosclerosis and cardiovascular disease. The theory was widely accepted among the medical and scientific communities for a prolonged period of time. All kinds of drugs were created and prescribed to reduce cholesterol levels.

Statin drugs, such as Lipitor, were designed to block the enzymes that are required to make cholesterol. It was believed that if we blocked the body's capacity to make cholesterol, then the problem would not continue.

So why is this all being disputed now?

1. The liver makes 80% of the body's cholesterol and for good reason. We require cholesterol for:

    1. Outer rim of the cell — required to regulate what goes in and out of the cell

    2. Bill — breaks down the fats that you digest; and allows you to absorb the good fats

    3. Hormones — all the steroid hormones: testosterone, estrogen, cortisol, aldosterone

    4. Vitamin D — required to make Vitamin D

    5. Insulation — the neurons in the brain require proper insulation to work and they need fat

    6. Absorption of fat based vitamins — A, D, E, K

    7. Acts as an anti-oxidant

    8. Contributes to bone formation — they would be hollow and brittle without it

    9. Cholesterol plaque is there to protect damaged arteries — a clogged artery is better than a ruptured one

    10. Oxidation of cholesterol is the 1st step by which cholesterol transforms into vitamin D3

    11. Cholesterol sulfate deficiency leads to glucose intolerance

12. Cholesterol is not only important to the brain but higher serum levels of cholesterol is correlated with higher cognitive function.[2]

Ancel Keys created the original study. He published a study that supposedly crossed over several countries, identifying that heart disease was associated with fat intake.

So what was the problem?

The problem was, as is often the case in pharmaceutical research, he evidently tossed out the data that did not fit with his hypothesis. Consequently, according to many, the original research crossed 22 countries but was reported as being based on only seven countries. The now infamous graph was based on Australia, Britain, Canada, Japan, Italy, US, however, the study[3] included Northern Europe (Finland, Netherlands), Southern Europe (Italy), Yugoslavia, Greece, and Japan.[4] In fact, the study became known as the Seven Countries Study.

No one seems to know why Keys only included six of the 22 countries in the graph, especially in consideration of the fact that when all 22 countries are combined, the same association between fat and heart disease occurs. So was he right?

Another interesting fact is that when Keys initially presented his study to a group at Mount Sinai Hospital in New York and then later the infamous presentation at the WHO, it was apparently met with skepticism and he left the conference before presenting all his data. The question is, if it was met with criticism and skepticism then, why is it so widely accepted as fact now? And, why do so many say the study was wrong?

A variety of factors were not taken into consideration...

1. What type of fat?

    o Today we know that omega 6s are pro-inflammatory, whereas

    o Omega 3s are anti-inflammatories

2. Were there other dietary components that played a stronger role?

3. What are the interactions between different dietary components, i.e. Vitamin D, K1, k2 and calcium?

4. What about toxins? Do different fats combine differently with different toxins, which would come up more recently?

5. What was the health condition of the people in the study?

6. How accurate were the sources of data?

So, let's actually take a look at the study and see what it really tells us:

1. Heart disease goes up when calories include a higher intake of animal fat.

2. Heart disease goes up when animal proteins take up a higher component of calories.

3. Heart disease goes up when a higher percent of calories come from animal fat.

In addition, higher rates of plant fats decreased the risk of heart disease; higher rates of plant proteins also decreased the risk of heart disease.

Vegetarians might respond with "see, we told you so". But the problem here is that it is still a correlational study *not* a study of cause and effect. This is a big challenge with a lot of "medical studies" because there is a big difference between correlation and causal studies.

This is so important that we are going to take a step aside and give you a good understanding of why correlational studies do *not* provide causal information.

To give you an example: There is a strong correlation between me getting up at sunrise; however, the sun does not get me up. What woke me up might be:

1. The sun (if the sun pours in through the windows and the light bothers my eyes)

2. The alarm clock

3. The dogs

4. Habit

5. A bad dream

6. The kids making noises

Any of these, or any combination, might contribute to waking me up. But I didn't say "wake up", I said "get up".

Now there may also be a correlation between me actually getting up and the sun rising. The cause may be I:

7. Have to go to the bathroom

8. Can't stand the sludge in my mouth

9. Have a bad taste in my mouth

10. Want to get a good start on the day

11. Want to get some time alone to:

    o   Go for a run

    o   Meditate

    o   Get some work done

12. Might be hungry

13. Can't stand just lying there doing nothing

So, while there is a correlation between me getting up with the sunrise, it is neither a factor in waking me up nor getting me up. Unfortunately, the misuse of words can easily lead people astray when they do not have clarity on what the terms actually mean.

Back to the study on cholesterol…it appears from the data that the countries with "the lowest rates of death from arteriosclerosis and degenerative heart disease" had suspiciously high rates of "death from other diseases of the heart". There is a clue there, let's keep looking.[5]

Another factor that needed to be checked is when they looked at deaths from everything other than heart disease, the pattern reversed:

- Fat was negatively associated with death

- Animal fat was negatively associated with death

- Animal protein was negatively associated with death

- Those participants with the higher percentage of carbohydrates in their calorie intake had the highest mortality rates

- In fact, in those countries where fats contribute to over 30% of the diet, people had the longest life expectancies!

So now non-vegetarians will say, "See, we told you so!"

Isn't that interesting…so how do we account for this? Let's examine two factors:

- Some of the countries chosen for the graph had poor coding methods, i.e. they dump a large number of heart disease deaths into the wrong categories.

- Apparently, "the amount of fat and protein available for consumption is an index of a country's development, industrially, nutritionally, medically, and no doubt in other respects as well."[6]

Taking this a step further, if fat consumption is correlated with the country's economic status and level of industrialization, you can bet they also have a lot more:

1. Processed foods

2. Pasteurized foods

3. Microwaved foods

4. Fast foods

5. Toxicity (food, environmental, etc.)

Do you think there might a relationship between all of these variables and heart disease?

Wait, let's learn from past mistakes and *not* jump to conclusions.

Let's take another look at Keye's research. In a paper entitled: *Human atherosclerosis and the diet*[7], Keyes wrote "from these animal experiments only, the most reasonable conclusion would be that the cholesterol content of human diets is unimportant in human atherosclerosis".

What? From the very man to whom we attribute the problem with diet cholesterol issue, claimed that it wasn't an issue?

He even made another comment in another paper: "The evidence—both from experiments and from field surveys—indicates that the cholesterol content, per se, of all natural diets has *NO* significant effect on either the serum cholesterol level or the development of atherosclerosis in man". (Page 182, Symposium on Atherosclerosis 1955.)[8]

So what physicians have been taught for the last sixty years is, in effect, false.

Cholesterol

The above research focused on fats in the body and from there, assumptions were made about cholesterol. Let's take a moment and understand what cholesterol actually is.

First, there are two major types of cholesterol:

- Unesterified or free cholesterol (UC)

61

- Esterified cholesterol (CE)

The majority of cholesterol in our diets is CE and it is *not* absorbed but is excreted by our gut in the stool. In order to be absorbed, it has to be "de-esterfied" and it has to compete with the UC, which is in vastly larger amounts and produced by the liver. Consequently, the body has made the majority of cholesterol in the body.

The body uses all kinds of fats for a variety of things in the body, as noted above but fats need to move to different places. Fats therefore require transport mechanisms to move.

Basically, cholesterol is required in the blood stream in order to carry different fat/lipid molecules and compounds. The guys that regulate the transportation of fats in the blood are called *apoproteins* and when these proteins are bound to fats/lipids, they are called *lipoproteins (A and B)* or *apolipoprotiens*. Fats move in the blood in lipoprotein vehicles.

These vehicles are made in a very specific way. They are surrounded by proteins and phospholipids on the outside with cholesterol "stents" holding the structure up. The triacylglycerols (TG) and cholesterol esters travel on the inside or attached to the outer membrane.

There are two major groups:

1. Apolipoproteins A (composed of alpha-helices which connect with alpha proteins) have higher density (and are associated with HDLs).

2. Apolipoprotines B (composed of beta pleated sheets which connect with beta proteins) have

lower density and are associated with VLDS, IDLs and LDLs.

What is important here is that:

- As the cholesterol concentration increases,

- The TG concentration decreases,

- As the lipoproteins go from large to small

Why? As the VLDLs become IDLs and then possibly LDLs, they have consequently become cholesterol rich.

The liver produces the VLDLs. We need them because they are important for transporting cholesterols back to the liver, as noted above.

Note: At one time they thought only the HDLs carried the cholesterols back to the liver but we now know that the LDLs do this, too. In fact, the LDLs carry more cholesterol back to the liver than the HDLs do. Wow! Did you get that?

The *bad* cholesterol does a better clean up job than the *good* cholesterol. Whoops, did they ever get that wrong!

But wait a minute. Don't get too excited. There can be a problem with LDLs.

Sometimes, under certain circumstances, the LDLs penetrate the arterial lining and cause a problem. Most cells in the body produce enough of their own cholesterol and consequently don't need more cholesterol delivered.

Now, let's view this from another angle. Most physicians will test you for:

- HDL (high density lipoprotein — claimed to be the good guys)

- LDL (low density lipoprotein — claimed to be the bad guys)

- TGs (triglyceride — not good)

But has your physician ever looked at the breakdown of these cholesterols?

1. HDL 2a and 2b: You want these to be high as they *extract* fats from arterial walls and prevent fats from adhering to the walls.

2. HDL 3: You want to be lower than HDL 2

3. LDL A: These are large and buoyant LDL and you want a good supply of these.

4. LDL B: These are predominantly the smaller and denser LDL. You don't want these to be high as they can lead to diabetes, high blood pressure, and arteriosclerosis.

5. LDL mixed

6. LDL R: This is the one that is associated with a bad diet.

7. LDL a: This is a good inflammatory marker and we want it to be low. We always have inflammation in the body as simply lying down and breathing is going to cause arterials to break. Inflammation occurs in order to resolve the breakage. But we want low, *not* high, levels of inflammation.

8. IDL: Intermediate density lipoprotein. In 1981, simple correlational analysis showed a positive correlation between IDL and LDL and a negative correlation with HDLs and coronary heart disease for men. [9] This is similar to an LDL but without the TG, i.e. it transports TG fats and cholesterols and can promote growth of atheroma.

9. Lp(a): Lipoprotein a consists of an LDL-like particle and controlled genetically; kidney function is important for clearing it.

10. VLDL 1,2: These are very large. They transport TGs to adipose and muscle cells (for energy, cellular maintenance, steroid creation, etc.). They also transport cholesterol from the gut to the liver. They release some of their TGs in the form of fatty acids as well as some of their surface phospholipids and consequently they shrink in size. Now the VLDL becomes an IDL, which may undergo further reduction and become LDLs. However, the liver cleans up most of the IDL particles (assuming it is working well).

When you start looking at all the different types of cholesterol, you find:

- Not all HDL is good (in fact it is important to make sure that HDL 2 is predominant over HDL 3)

- Not all LDL is bad (in fact you want LDL A; LDL A is a good non-oxidized cholesterol where LDL B is an oxidized cholesterol)

- LDLs do more clean up than HDLs

So what do you need in order to get a proper reading of your cholesterol counts, a spec analysis?

Before we go any further, here is a quote from Dr. Mercola:

"The media and health experts have been giving out massive misinformation about cholesterol. High cholesterol and high-fat diets are really *not* the cause of heart disease. Statistical lies, flawed science, and cherry-picked data are perpetuating cholesterol myths that may be harming your health. The most effective way to optimize your cholesterol profile and prevent heart disease is via diet and exercise, *not* statin drugs. The high-cholesterol/heart disease myth began more than 100 years ago when a German pathologist theorized that cholesterol led to development of plaques in your arteries."[10]

But if it is not dietary cholesterol that is causing plaque and heart disease, what is causing it? Let's continue.

SIX

If dietary cholesterol is not the problem, what is?

There are several answers to this question, so let's go one by one. First off, just to make things really easy for everyone, here is a short list of some of the worst foods for your heart:

Candy

Chocolate (either be the best thing for your heart or the worst. See my book: *The Chocolate Controversy: the bad, the mediocre and the awesome.*

- Deep dish pepperoni pizza
- Deep fried chicken
- Deli meats
- Donuts
- Fast foods
- Gravy slathered fries
- Ice cream

To extend the list, we could be more general and say:

- Anything that has processed sugars
  - Baking
  - Pizzas
  - Candies
  - Junk food

- o   Fast food
- Anything that has processed fats
  - o   Deep fried anything
  - o   Breaded meats and vegetables
  - o   Margarines and other artificial butters
  - o   Again much baking and pizzas
  - o   Burgers and other fast foods
  - o   Milk shakes
  - o   Pasta sauces and salad dressings
  - o   Potato chips and the dips
- Anything that has synthetic chemicals
  - o   Okay so practically everything above +
  - o   Deli meats
  - o   Sausages, sausage roles, etc.
- Anything that is GMO
- Most carbonated and/or energy drinks

Some may claim that red meat is bad for the heart. I suggest that if it is not injected with antibiotics and growth hormones and it is still grazed then it can be beneficial, so find a store that promotes good healthy red meats.

But we all know this, so let's look at some details and find out what is really going on.

First, we know that when the arteries are blocked, regardless of the reason:

1. This puts pressure on the heart

2. Heart has to compensate for lack of vasodilation of the arteries

3. Oxygen isn't getting to all the necessary parts of the body

4. Toxins are not being removed, because the blood is not moving

5. Extra pressure is being put on the kidneys (responsible for keeping the blood thin enough)

What can affect the arteries so that the blood is restricted?

1. Many people will simply write this off as "inflammation" and they may be right but if we are going to get to the bottom of this problem, we need to understand what is causing the inflammation.

2. Low levels of nitric oxide — required for vasodilation. Remember, arteries have smooth muscles lining them so that they can expand and contract both allowing the blood flow and pushing the blood flow.

3. Low levels of Vitamin K2 (we also have K1 and K3 (Synthetic)). K2 is made by the bacteria in your gut and goes straight to the blood vessels, bones and other tissues as opposed to going through your liver. But even K2 can be further broken down:

   i) MK-4 (menaquinone-4) which is found in butter, egg yolks, and animal based foods

ii) MK-7 (menaquinone-7) a longer chain found in fermented foods (one of the many reasons fermented foods are so good for you)

iii) Note: if you are buying K2 as a supplement, you want the MK-7 version because:

1. It is made from fermented products

2. It stays in your body longer

3. It has a longer half life

4. Low levels of Vitamin D3, which is required to create more K2-dependent proteins that move calcium around in the body. Vitamin D3 and K2 work in a wonderful interdependent dance but the more Vitamin D you have, the more K2 you need.

5. Too much calcium: What? You have always been told to take calcium supplements to strengthen your bones. However, more calcium is "correlated" with a higher incidence of heart attacks and strokes. Why? Because if there is insufficient Vitamin D and K2, the calcium doesn't go where it needs to and can end up causing calcification on the arterial lining. Now foods typically high in calcium are also high in Vitamin K2. That's a not only a blessing but it also means we must look to the foods rather than the supplements.

6. Too little magnesium: You may have heard that magnesium is required for over 380 functions in every cell. It is also required for the proper function of calcium. Vitamin K2 and magnesium

complement one another *and* magnesium helps to lower blood pressure. Magnesium is required for:

o   Production of ATP/fuel in every cell

o   Dilates/relaxes blood vessels

o   Prevents spasm in your heart muscle

o   Prevents spasm in your blood vessels walls

o   Counteracts the action of calcium – which increases spasm in the heart muscle – both are required

o   Dissolves blood clots

o   Prevents arrhythmia

o   Acts as an anti-oxidant (eliminates free radicals) at the site of an injury

o   Regulation of blood sugar levels

Typically, we require twice as much magnesium as we do calcium.

SEVEN

Nutrients for the heart

Now that you have learned what a hard working organ the heart is. You can guess that it needs a lot of nutrients to keep it going. It is a difficult process to identify exactly what nutrients we require for the heart, because just produce to the ATP/fuel we need:

- The Krebs cycle – the byproducts are required for
- The electron transfer chain (ETC)
- Which produces the ATP

So before we look at the heart in general, let's briefly go over what it takes to make fuel for the heart cell. The Krebs cycle requires:

- Proteins, carbs and fat are metabolized into Acetyl Coenzyme A
- Carbs and sugars are metabolized to glucose
- Glucose is metabolized into pyruvic acid and then into acetyl coenzyme A
- Citric acid, malic acid, fumaric acid, succinic acid, pyruvic acid, pantothenic acid, alpha-ketoglutaric acid (which produces L-glutamine), lipoic acid
- Vitamins B1, B2, B3, B5
- Magnesium, phosphorus, manganese, iron, sulfur[1]

72

Then the ETC requires:

- CoQ10
- Iron
- Copper
- Phosphorus [2]

All that just to create the ATP fuel for every cell! An important item to note is that every cell in the body requires these nutrients in order to make fuel/ATP. Every cell in the body, including heart cells, has numerous "organelles" or cell organs. The following is a list of the basic components of any given cell:

- Cell membrane
- Centrosome
- Cytoskeleton
- Cytosol (this is actually the fluid that fills the cell)
- Golgi apparatus
- Lysosomes
- Mitochondria
- Nucleolus
- Nucleus
- Ribosome
- Rough endoplasmic reticulum
- Smooth endoplasmic reticulum
- Vacuole
- Vesicle

As you can well imagine, every cell in the body requires nutrients to make all of these components and:

- The fuel
- The tools
- The enzymes
- The nutrients…

to make all of these different organelles.

Don't worry; we are not going to go through all of that. Just remember, when we are talking about the nutrients required by a heart cell or the heart as an organ, we are just providing the most superficial list. There is a lot more going on "than meets the eye", as the old saying goes.

Now in general, we can say that the heart requires:

1. *Omega 3 fatty acids* — these are the ones associated with the anti-inflammatory system and include:

   - alpha linolenic acid (ALA)
   - eicopentaenoic acid (EPA)
   - docosahexaenoic acid (DHA)

Omega 3s are found in the following foods:

- 100% pure chocolate
- Salmon (be careful of the mercury)
- Ground flaxseed (we don't have the enzymes to break down the seed so make sure they are ground)

74

- Hemp seed

- Salba or chia seed

- Oatmeal

- Beans (black beans or kidney beans)

- Nuts: walnuts, almonds

- Nut and seed oils (almond, sesame, etc.). Olive oil has typically lost its omega 3s within six months after processing, and too many companies have been caught combining their olive oil with cheaper oils.

2. *CoQ10* — required in every cell of the body and for different purposes (see Chapter 8 for more information).

   1. CoQ10 is the "limiting factor" to make ATP, the fuel for any cell in the body.

      - An example of a limiting factor is if I ask you to make pancakes for a 100 people and give you an unlimited supply of flour, milk, and baking powder but only one egg, your one egg is the limiting factor.

   2. One of the many problems with statin drugs is that they not only prevent the body from making cholesterol but also prevent the body from making CoQ10.

   3. CoQ10 is also an anti-oxidant.

4. The challenge with CoQ10, is that like many other compounds, you can get different versions of it: ubiquinol or ubiquinone. Some research claims that different forms are better at different ages. We will explore that in Chapter 8.

5. CoQ10 is found in the following foods:

- Beef
- Soy products (be careful it is not GMO)
- Sardines
- Mackerel

3. *Vitamin D3* — although it is not really a hormone, it is not a vitamin. While we can take Vitamin D3 as a supplement, it is far better to make it in the skin, as the byproducts of making Vitamin D3 are anti-carcinogens.

4. *Vitamin K1 and K2* — Did you know that Vitamin K comes in different forms and that each does something different?

1. Vitamin K1 (phylloquinone) which is found in green vegetables, helps regulate healthy blood clotting; and helps your bones retain calcium

2. Vitamin K2 (menaquinone) is found in fermented foods and goes directly to vessel walls, bones and various tissues but is not metabolized by the liver. Vitamin K2 prevents calcification of blood vessels, which is very important. A significant component of arterial plaque actually consists of calcium

deposits (atherosclerosis) thus causing "hardening of the arteries". K2 is found in the following foods:

- Dried and fresh herbs:
    o Basil
    o Sage
    o Thyme
    o Parsley
    o Coriander
    o Marjoram
    o Oregano
- And spices:
    o Chili powder
    o Curry
    o Paprika
    o Cayenne pepper
- Leafy vegetables:
    o Kale
    o Dandelion
    o Collards
    o Cress
    o Spinach
    o Turnip
    o Mustard greens
    o Beet greens
    o Swiss chard
    o Onions, especially spring onions
    o Brussel sprouts, Broccoli, cabbage
    o Asparagus
    o Pickled cucumber

3. *Vitamin K3 (menadione).* Yes, there is actually another form of Vitamin K but there appears to be confusion about it. The synthetic form of Vitamin K is man-made and not recommended. Note: There is an intricate dance between calcium, Vitamin D3, K1, and K2 (and Vitamin K3 appears to convert K1 into K2 in mice; some claim that vitamin K3 is made in the intestines from K1).

5. *Quercetin* — A plant-derived flavonoid that contains anti-inflammatory properties and is found in apples. Remember the old saying "an apple a day keeps the doctor away"? Apparently, there is a lot of truth to that.

   a. Note: New studies show that an apple a day is as potent as taking a statin drug.

   b. Note: Walking every day is also as potent as taking a statin drug.

6. *Folate or Folic acid or Vitamin M or Vitamin B9.* Folate helps to regulate homocysteine, an amino acid. Current belief holds that when homocysteine is too high you are at risk for heart attacks, vascular disease and strokes. Folate is found in abundance in:

   1. Green leafy vegetables: The highest concentration found in:
      - Spinach
      - Asparagus
      - Brussel sprouts
      - Mom told you to eat your vegetables!

2. Fruits
3. Nuts
4. Beans
5. Peas
6. Dairy products
7. Poultry
8. Meat
9. Eggs
10. Seafood
11. Grains

7. *Monounsaturated fats found in:*
   - 100% pure chocolate
   - Avocados
   - Pecans
   - Good, expensive olive oil (most olive oil is a scam)

8. *L-carnitine* – an amino acid found in almost all of our cells but is associated with the heart and is found in:
   - Avocados
   - Fermented soy foods
   - Animal protein

9. *L-arginine* – another amino acid that is important for the vascular system because it is the precursor to nitric oxide (NO). NO is required to promote vasodilation, the expansion or relaxation of the arteries. As the arteries expand and contract they push the oxygenated blood through your body. If the arteries cannot expand and contract – more

pressure is put onto the heart to push the blood.[3] Foods high in arginine include:

- Seeds: sesame, sesame flour
- Gelatins
- Soy protein isolate
- Peanut flour
- Crustaceans: crab, lobster, shrimp
- Seaweed, spirulina
- Spinach
- Game meat
- Chicken

10. **Lycopene** — Gives tomatoes their colour. Lycopene increases the levels of super oxide dismutase (SOD) an important anti-oxidant and helps to reduce blood pressure and C-reactive protein (CRP), which is a marker used to indicate cardiac inflammation, although it is a marker for any acute phase inflammation. Note: We do not have the enzymes to break down the cellular membrane of tomatoes so make sure your tomatoes are cooked

11. **Magnesium** — An important mineral for the body and required for over 380 basic cell functions in every cell of the body. Magnesium is found in:

- 100% pure chocolate
- Walnuts
- Spinach
- Used to be broccoli but not anymore

12. *Polyphenols*—While there are thousands of this phytonutrient, they typically work as an anti-oxidant but also helps to keep nitric oxide levels up. Nitric oxide is used to promote vasodilation/relaxation in the arteries thus allowing blood pressure to reduce. When the arteries can expand and contract like they are supposed to, using the smooth muscle found in lining of the artery, this takes the pressure off the heart to push the blood. They are found in:

- 100% pure chocolate
- Blueberries
- Raspberries
- Strawberries (be careful because strawberries absorb more toxins than any other food)

13. *Allicin*—The main active ingredient in garlic. Rooms full of studies have been done on garlic.

- Allicin produces hydrogen sulfide, which signals blood vessels to relax, increases blood flow and a variety of other functions.
- To get the most out of garlic, smash it, scoop and swallow without chewing. Cardio Research Center confirmed this at the Connecticut University School of Medicine.[4]

14. *Reservatrol*—is a good anti-oxidant that also promotes nitric oxide production and is found in:

81

- 100% pure chocolate
- Organic red wine

15. *Grapefruits* — are rich in polyphenols and anti-oxidants and help to lower LDLs; red grapefruits even lower triglycerides (TGs), a type of fat thought to harden arteries.

Did you notice how often 100% pure chocolate came up? Sounds good, doesn't it? We will look into this further in Chapter 10.

If we ate in accordance with the above list, we would have a pretty good healthy style of eating and living. (Notice I did not use the word "diet".)

What if we are getting all these nutrients in our diet? Shouldn't we have a good strong heart?

Perhaps, but there are also many other factors that can destroy these nutrients.

The question is, what happens if we are deficient in any given nutrients? Good questions.

EIGHT

CoQ10 – Ubiquinone versus Ubiquinol

What is CoQ10?

How do we make CoQ10?

Where do we use CoQ10?

What kind of CoQ10 do we need?

What depletes it?

Let's take a look…

What is CoQ10?

CoQ10 is also known as Coenzyme Q 10, ubiquione (fully oxidized), ubidecarenone, and ubiquinol (the reduced form). The "Q" refers to the Quinone chemical group and the number "10" refers to the number of isoprenyl chemical sub-units in its tail.

Apart from all that chemistry, it is a fat-soluble compound that functions as:

- An anti-oxidant protecting against DNA damage

- Required for Vitamin E to act an anti-oxidant

- A vitamin like compound

- The limiting factor in making ATP/fuel in every cell

Let's focus on the last item first, the "limiting factor" in making ATP/fuel. This is the primary function of CoQ10, so what does that mean?

83

Every cell in the body requires ATP/fuel. The amount of ATP required by a given cell is correlated with the number of mitochondria in the cell, which makes sense considering that the mitochondria make the ATP.

The organs requiring the most ATP/fuel and therefore have the most mitochondria in the cells are:

- Heart
- Liver
- Kidneys

To give you an idea of the numbers we are looking at—the average cell requires about 500 mitochondria, whereas a heart cell requires between 1000 - 2500 mitochondria in order to produce enough fuel to keep going.

We also said CoQ10 was the "limiting factor" in making this required fuel. In Chapter Six, we provided the example of a limiting factor:

If I ask you to make pancakes for a 100 people and give you an unlimited supply of flour, milk, and baking powder, but only one egg—your one egg is the limiting factor.

What has that got to do with making ATP/fuel?

How do we make CoQ10?

CoQ10 shares the same biological pathway as cholesterol. Cholesterol is made in the "Mevalonate Pathway". Statin drugs block the HMG-CoA reductase enzyme in the Mevalonate Pathway, which blocks the production of both cholesterol and CoQ10.

Other drugs like beta-blockers and hypertension medications can also block the production of CoQ10.

Where do we use CoQ10?

How does this organelle, the mitochondria, make this fuel? Let's quickly look at the process of making ATP.

Again, we addressed the complex process of making ATP/fuel in Chapter Six. Let's explore this a little bit further.

There are 3 major processes required to make ATP:

- Glycolysis
- Krebs cycle aka citric acid cycle
- Electron transfer chain aka ETC

Glycolysis is the term given to the ten-step, enzyme catalyzed, metabolic pathways that converts glucose (yes we need sugar!) into pyruvate.

Various monosaccharides or sugars can be utilized in this pathway, i.e. fructose or galactose, although their preparation for entry into the pathway is slightly different. If there is insufficient sugar then the body has additional means by which it can organize either fatty acids or proteins to begin the next step.

The process occurs in virtually all organisms, both aerobic (those that require oxygen) and anaerobic (those that don't require oxygen).

The *Krebs cycle* is a series of ten basic chemical reactions, supported by numerous other chemical reactions, and used by all aerobic organisms to make the by-products that are utilized to make ATP.

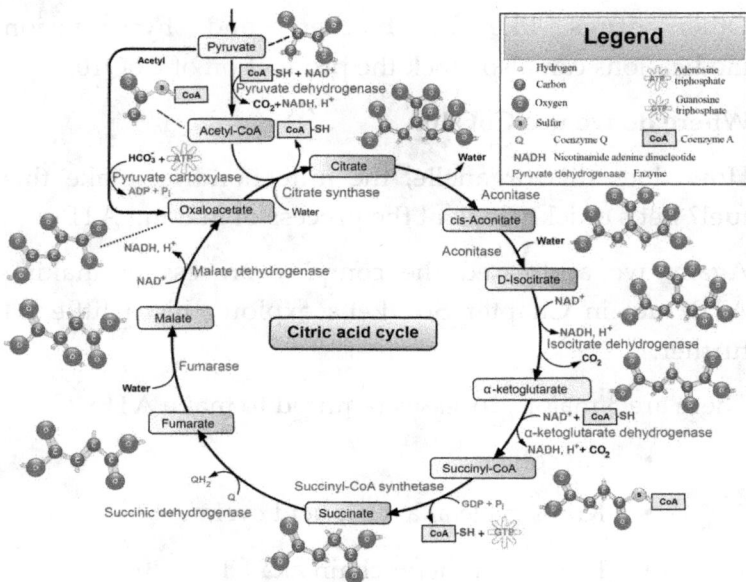

The byproducts of the Krebs cycle than go into the ETC:

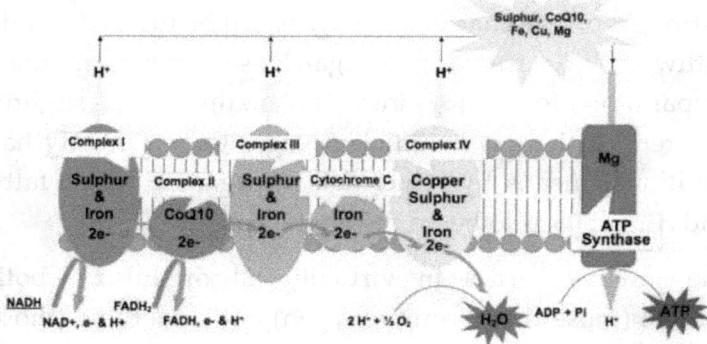

In the **ETC**, CoQ10 plays the role of transferring electrons from the "Enzyme Complex I and Enzyme Complex II to Complex III".[2]

What is interesting is that in current research, it appears that "vitamin K2 co-functions in this role with CoQ10".[3]

Nutrients that the ETC requires are:

- Phosphorous
- Copper
- Iron
- Manganese
- CoQ10

Okay, so we have identified what CoQ10 is and how we make it. Now, we have to identify which kind we need. There are different types of CoQ10 as well? Yup.

What kind of CoQ10 do we need?

There is controversy over which type of CoQ10, ubiquinone, and ubiquinol, is most utilized. Some studies claim that as you age, your capacity to convert ubiquinone to ubiquinol (the active anti-oxidant version) decreases.

Thus, the conclusion is that the older you get the more you need to supplement with ubiquinol increases. Dr. Mercola sites studies indicating that ubiquinol is more important the older you get. [4]

Usana™ will quote studies indicating that there isn't any difference in the form but rather in the formulization, i.e. using oil versus powder. [5]

A third party, Dr. Stephen Sinatra, says there is no data to support the claims that one is absorbed better than the other.[6]

What depletes CoQ10?

The biggest items that deplete CoQ10 are statin drugs. As noted earlier, statin drugs are well known for blocking the enzyme that prevents the body from producing CoQ10. Other drugs block and/or deplete CoQ10 as well.

According to the University of Maryland the following drugs are known to deplete CoQ10:

Anti-depressant drugs: TCAs

1. Amitriptyline:

   - Elavil
   - Vanatrip

2. Amoxapine

   - Asendin

3. Clomipramine

   - Anafranil

4. Desipranine

   - Norpramin

5. Doxepin

   - Sinequan oral
   - Zonalon topical cream

6. Imipramine

   - Tofranil – PM
   - Tofranil

7. Nortiptyline

- Aventyl
- Pamelor

8. Protriptyline

   - Vivactil

9. Trimipramine

   - Surmonti

Cholesterol lowering drugs:

1. Fibric acid Derivatives

   - Gemifibrozil: Lopid

2. HMG-CoA reductase inhibitors (Statins)

   - Atorvastatin: Lipitor

3. Fluvastatin: Lescol; Lescol XL

4. Lovastatin: Mevacor

5. Pravastatin: Pravachol

6. Simvastatin: Zocor

Diabetic drugs: Sulfonylureas

1. Acetohexamide: Dymelor

2. Chlorpropamide: Diabineses

3. Glipzide: Glucotrol, Glucotrol XL

4. Glyburide:

   - DiaBeta
   - Glynase Pres Tab
   - Micronase

5. Tolazamide: Tolinase

6. Tolbutamide: Orinase, Tol-Tab

Diuretics: Thiazide diuretics

1. Chlorothiazide: Diuril

   - Hydrochlorothiazide:
   - Aquazide
   - Esidrix
   - Ezide
   - Hydrocot
   - HydroDIURIL
   - Microzide
   - Oretic

2. Indapamide: Lozol

3. Methyclothiazide: Aquatensen; Enduron

4. Metolazone: Mykrox; Zaroxolyn

Heart drugs:

1. Alpha2 – Adrenergic Agonists

   - Clonidine
     o Catapress-TTS Transdermal
     o Catapres Oral
     o Duraclon
   - Methyladopa
     o Aldomet
   - Guanfacine
     o Tenex
   - Guanabenz
     o Wytensin

2. Beta Blockers

- Acebutolol: Sectral
- Atenolol: Tenormin
- Betaxolol: Betoptic, Betoptic S, Kerlone
- Bisoprolol: Cartrol Oral, Ocupress Ophthalmic
- Celiprolol: Celol
- Esmolol: Brevibloc
- Labetalol: Normodyne, Trandate
- Levobetaxolol: Betaxon
- Levobunolol: Betagan
- Metipranolol: Optipranolol
  - Metoprolol: Lopressor, Toprol XL
  - Nadolol: Corgard
  - Penbutolol: Levatol
  - Pindolol: Visken
  - Propranolol: Inderal, Inderal LA
  - Sotalol: Betapace AF, Betapace
  - Timolol:
    - Betimol
    - Blocadren
    - Timoptic-XE
    - Timoptic
    - Timoptic OcuDose

3. Vasodilators:

- Hydralazine: Apresoline

Psychotherapeutic drugs:

1. Phenothiazine derivatives

2. Thioxanthene derivatives[7]

It is scary that in 1972, both Littamu and Folkers both identified a deficiency of CoQ10 in people with heart disease. Since that time, there have been numerous clinical studies establishing the same issue.

Yet, all these drugs are known to further deplete CoQ10. And it is only in the last couple of years that cardiologists have suggested to the patients prescribed statin drugs, that they supplement their diet with CoQ10. But what about all the other patients receiving medications that deplete CoQ10?

In another book I wrote called, *Your Vital Liver*, I detail all of the different drugs that are prescribed today, and all the nutrients that these drugs deplete.

You would think that MDs would have both a moral and a legal obligation to know this information and inform their clients. But there is another whole issue that we have not even addressed yet.

NINE

Vitamin D3

Most people have heard that we need Vitamin D3 but don't know...

- Why D3 as opposed to the other Ds?
- How do I make it?
- What does it do for me?
- What happens if I am deficient?
- What does it do for the heart?
- Do I really need supplements?
- How do I know if it is a good supplement?

Before we look at answering these questions, let's clarify something. Vitamin D operates more like a steroid hormone (it travels through the body) than a vitamin.

Why Vitamin D3?

Vitamin D is a group of secosteroids:

- **Vitamin D2**: Ergocalcifoer — made by plants; liver converts D2 into 25-hydroxyergocalciferol

- **Vitamin D3:** Cholecalciferol — 87% more effective than D2; can be synthesized through the skin and from cholesterol, if there is sufficient sun; liver converts D3 into calcidiol in the liver; kidney converts calcidiol into calcitriol

- **Calcitriol:** circulates in the blood as a hormone and regulates the concentration of calcium and phosphate

What does it do for me?

Vitamin D3 is the most important of the compounds and is involved in the following:

- Absorption of calcium, iron, magnesium, phosphate and zinc

- Bone health — deficiency: bones become thin, brittle, misshapen, osteomalacia, osteoporosis

- Required for general growth

- Required for brain development

- Required for the immune system

- Required to help the kidneys regulate blood pressure

- Required to help regulate the blood sugar levels in the pancreas

- Required for neuro-muscle function

- Required for healthy respiratory function

- Impacts on about 3000 of your 25,000 genes

- Prevent 16 types of cancer

  o Increases self-destruction of mutated cells

  o Reduces the spread/reproduction of cancer cells

  o Causes cells to become differentiated (cancer cells are usually undifferentiated)

- o Reduces the growth of new blood vessels (angiogenesis) with tumors [1,2]

As noted in prior chapters, Vitamin D3 works in an intricate dance with Vitamin K2.

What happens if I am deficient?

Deficiency is now linked to:

- Alter the regulatory function of the parathyroid (which also regulates calcium in the blood)

- Back pain (chronic low back pain)

- Bone dysfunction (osteopenia, osteoporosis, osteomalacia)

- Cancer

- Cognitive function declines

- Depression

- Diabetes/insulin resistance (60% have a deficiency)

- Impaired immune function

- Kidney dysfunction

- Macular degeneration

- Muscle weakness [3]

An important factor here is that we can be deficient because it is being absorbed by fat cells, which prevents it from circulating.

What does it do for the heart?

Dr. Michos, Assistant Professor of Medicine at John Hopkins Hospital, Cardiology Division, researchers the impact of Vitamin D on the heart and has found that increased levels of Vitamin D lower the risk of cardiovascular disease. She has found that Vitamin D helps to regulate blood pressure through the kidneys.

But is there anything else that can help the heart? Let's keep looking.

TEN

The chocolate controversy

Most people today have heard how good real chocolate is for them. Here is a short review of some of the highlights (Note: For more in-depth information, please read my book, *The Chocolate Controversy: the bad, the mediocre and the awesome*).[1]

Like any fruit or vegetable, the seed of the cocoa fruit is the most nutrient dense. The reason so much research has been done on chocolate is that the seed has over 1200 molecules, with over 300 nutrients in significant amount.

These nutrients include:

- Amino acids:
  - o Arginine
  - o Phenylalanine
  - o Taurine
  - o Tyramine
  - o Tryptophan

- Fatty acids:
  - o Stearic acids
  - o Palmitic acids
  - o Capric acid
  - o Myristic acid
  - o Arachidic acid
  - o Lauric acid

- o Oleic acid
- o Linoleic acid

- Fibre:

  - o Soluble
  - o Non-soluble

- Alkalizing minerals:

  - o Calcium
  - o Chromium
  - o Iron
  - o Manganese
  - o Magnesium
  - o Phosphorous
  - o Zinc

- Vitamins

  - o Vitamin A
  - o B Vitamins: B1, B2, B3, B5, B6
  - o Vitamin C
  - o Vitamins K1 and K2

- Neurotransmitters

  - o Anandamide (also converts to the arachidonic acid cycle)
  - o Dopamine

- Endorphins:

  - o Opiod peptides

- Anti-depressants

  - o MAOIs (Pharmaceuticals have tried to replicate)

- Anti-oxidants (Powerful Polyphenols)

  o Epicatechins
  o Procynandins
  o (Note: There are thousands of anti-oxidants and most are damaged by heat so whenever they are pasteurized, have boiling water poured on them, are boiled in water, or are in any way heated – you lose them.)

- Phytonutrients

  o Theobromine (diuretic, vasodilator)

- Supports production of:

  o Glutathione
  o Nitric oxide

- And much more

So when we look at this list, some really important nutrients stand out for the heart:

- Anti-oxidants

- Glutathione

- Minerals: magnesium, calcium

- Vasodilators: nitric oxide and theobromine

- Vitamins: B1, B2, B3

Because of the above, chocolate ends up being incredibly beneficial to the heart:

- Increases vascular vasodilation/relaxation
- Provides the vitamins and alkalizing minerals necessary for the heart

- Provides the anti-oxidants and anti-inflammatories for the heart and vascular system

Wow, junk chocolate can be so bad for you but good chocolate can be so good for you!

ELEVEN

Your heart and your gut

What? Your gut can affect your heart?

In the past year, there has been a huge amount of focus on the gut's microbiota, thanks to new technology that is able to profile it more effectively.

We know that there are over 1000 different types of gut bacteria in the small and large intestine. We know that most of it comes from about 40-50 species. We know that we have more "good" bacteria in the large intestine than we have cells in the whole body. We know that the "good" bacteria is immensely important to:

- Our immune system

- Preventing the "bad" gut pathogens from taking over

- Protecting the mucosal membrane of the gut

- Providing nutrients that we require

The gut microbiota has now been identified as being associated with a large number of issues throughout the body, from depression to schizophrenia to Parkinson's disease to liver issues to diabetes.

The microbiota is now recognized as being associated with various chronic diseases including elevated cholesterol[1]and coronary heart disease.[2] One study suggests that excessive consumption of red meat can alter the levels/ratios of the microbiota.[3]

What we are finding out now is that not only do our gut microbiota do a lot more than what was previously thought, but that the balance/ratios of different groups has a huge impact on our physiology.

There are a wide variety of issues that need to be taken into consideration:

- The types of microbiota
- The numbers of microbiota
- The dominance of various types and groups of microbiota
- What their byproducts are
- What they feed off
- What the byproducts are from their feeding off fibers
- How they interact with fermented foods
- What kinds of immune cells they provoke in us
- How they regulate our inflammatory system
- Where they "live" in our gut mucosa
- What nerves they stimulate

All these factors and more can contribute to our good health and to our lack of good health. They can impact our cardiovascular and liver health. They can affect our cholesterol levels and blood pressure.

Most of the research in this area is new and still unfolding but it is powerful. It reinforces our need to support our gut health. Which then can contribute to and regulate our heart health.

TWELVE

Your heart and your teeth

I bet you didn't expect that your teeth have something to do with your gut, and your heart.

Dr. Weston Price was a dentist (1870 – 1948) who explored the world searching for the connection between nutrition, dental and physical health. In addition to being a devout researcher, he founded the National Dental Association as a research institute, which later became the research component of the American Dentist Association.

His conclusions, in his book, *Nutrition and Physical Degeneration* (1939), were that flour, sugar, and modern fats cause nutritional deficiencies that are a cause of numerous dental and health issues.

Can you believe that as far back as 1930, Dr. Price published a paper in the Journal of the American Dental Society, stating that nutrients like Vitamin A and Vitamin D fluctuated in buttermilk throughout the year? During the winter and dry summer months they significantly declined.

Note: If you want to read further about his work with the Mayo Clinic in the early part of the 1900s, go to: http://www.westonaprice.org/dentistry/root-canal-dangers

He took this a step further and graphed the number of deaths from heart attacks in the local hospitals and found that there was an inverse correlation between when the nutrients in the butter were low and deaths were high.

Today, we know that both nutrients are important for mineral absorption *and* support endocrine (hormone) function, *and* protect against inflammation, *and* Vitamin A is needed to convert cholesterol into steroid hormones, *and* that it is depleted with stress.[1]

How does Dr. Weston Price's understanding of teeth and what dentists are taught today differ?

Today dentists are taught that a tooth has 1 – 4 canals.

Dr. Weston identified as many as 75 separate accessary canals in a single tooth. These accessory canals, that dentists cannot reach, are the playground for both necrotic tissue (dead cells) but also hundreds of bacteria.

These bacteria can be toxic in and of themselves, or they can produce toxic byproducts. DNA studies have confirmed 83 different anaerobic bacteria. Root canals contain 53 different species. Common dangerous ones that occurred more than 5% of the time included:

- Capnocytophaga ochracea
- Fusobacterium nucleatum
- Gemella morbillorum
- Leptotrichia buccalis
- Porphyromonas gingivalis

How does this connect with the heart?

- Four of the above five, affect the heart

- Three of the above five, affect the nerves

- Two of the above five, affect the kidneys

105

- Two of the above five, affect the brain

- One of the above five affects the sinus cavities

So much for "safe" or "clean" root canals! Not only can these tubes not be cleaned but when tested, the "approximately 400 percent more bacteria were found in the blood surrounding the root canal tooth than were in the tooth itself. It seems that the tooth is the incubator".[2]

Another study found that of the top eight bacteria found in the blood adjacent to root canals teeth:

- Five affect the heart

- Five affect the nervous system

- Two affect the kidneys

- Two affect the liver

- One affects the brain sinus

We can understand why these bacteria found in the tooth, or in the root canal, can be found throughout the body. They travel in the blood.

Streptococcus mutants were found in 92% of the blood samples. Cause? Pneumonia, sinusitis, otitis media, meningitis, tooth decay. Streptococcus mitis was found 92% of the time and it attacks the heart and red blood cells.

It is unlikely that your dentist was taught all of this information but even if she or he was taught there is nothing that can be done to clean out the bacteria.

You may ask, why not just give antibiotics? Let's look at what happens when we provide antibiotics.

Most antibiotics are "bactericidal" meaning they don't just nicely kill bacteria but rather the bacterium explodes into fragments. For most bacteria, each of these fragments is a lipopolysaccharide and an endotoxin.

Exotoxins are the chemicals released from the bacteria whereas endotoxins are the toxic fragments of the original bacteria. So we can have a huge number of different types of bacteria and of any given type in each tooth. All of these could explode into hundreds or thousands of endotoxic pieces from just one capsule of a broad-spectrum antibiotic. And don't forget all the good bacteria they destroy in the process.

The immune system would have an extremely difficult time dealing with all of this.[3]

Are there any other issues with the teeth? They are called amalgams or the old-style fillings, which are not only full of mercury but also all kinds of other toxins.

With regard to mercury, here are a few facts. One thousand milligrams of mercury is 1 million times more mercury than found in contaminated seafood. It is by far the most toxic of any of the toxic metals such as aluminum, lead, arsenic, or cadmium.

- Amalgams slowly release a mercury vapor.

- When you chew or drink something hot – vapors are released.

- Vapors are absorbed into all your blood vessels in your mouth.

- This leads to excess oxidation leading to free radicals, inflammation, and decreased immune response.

- It damages the neurological system (Alzheimer's, Parkinson's, nerve damage and other nerve disorders).

- Mercury damages bones.

- Damages the endocrine (hormone) system.

- Damages the lining of the blood vessels.

- Liver produces more cholesterol to patch those damaged/bleeding blood vessels so you don't bleed to death.

- Overwhelms the liver with the need for detoxification.

Why don't dentists know this? The answer is that they are taught that the mercury in amalgams is bound with the other metals (which are toxic as well) and consequently doesn't leak. Yet the mercury vapor can be measured at the top of a tooth's root.

One of the body's anti-oxidants/enzymes, called catalase converts the mercury vapor into the Hg2plus form, which is extremely toxic. This gets trapped inside cells and we are still trying to find ways to get it removed.

Amalgams have other heavy toxic metals as well, such as:

- Mercury

- Silver

- Tin

- Zinc

- Copper

Why is the use of mercury in dental amalgam still allowed? Dentists benefit in the short term by being able to provide cheap fillings to those who can't afford healthy ones. The big pharmaceutical companies benefit because of all the disorders that result from its use.

Yet, amalgams have been banned in Denmark, Japan, Norway, Russia, and Sweden.[4,5,6]

Thankfully, the UN Treaty in January 2013 now requires countries to phase down the use of dental amalgams.[7]

However, if you have ever had amalgams, the mercury and other toxic metals may be hiding out in various tissues, and in particular fat cells, in the body. As noted above, these metals, and in particular the mercury, can damage blood vessels and the heart.

Ultimately, your body may be creating cardiovascular issues because of:

- Bacteria found in the teeth

- Bacteria found in the root canals

- Mercury in the amalgams

- Other toxic metals found in amalgam

Based on this information, we can safely conclude that your teeth might be causing or contributing to your cardiovascular issues.

THIRTEEN

Your heart and your mind

Your mind, whatever and wherever it resides, is what we think of as the seat of your thoughts and your emotions. When either your thoughts and/or your emotions are in conflict, they can affect your heart.

There is a direct connection between both psychological stress and gut stress *and* your adrenal glands. Your adrenal glands are the primary stress regulators. They respond to stress with the fight/flight response by shutting down the digestive system and sending all the energy to the peripheral muscles of the body to prepare for either fight or flight.

Our systems were designed to engage in a fight/flight response once in a while with a lot of time in-between to recover. Unfortunately, our western society has learned to live on adrenaline. As the adrenals produce adrenaline (epinephrine) and nor-adrenaline (nor-epinephrine), they keep the system pumped and allow us to keep going.

Like any other organ or system, if they are pushed too hard and/or for too long, they wear out. They also take a lot of nutrients from the body to function. They need nutrients to create all the different hormones and other factors that they both create and synthesize, and produce and secrete. For instance, how much ATP/energy do they need to create all the hormones they produce? During hyper-activity they have to regulate blood sugars for optimal use. They have to re-organize the energy usage in the body, which involves your immune and inflammatory systems, the temperature regulation of the body, and more.

If cortisol levels are too high for too long, we see:

- Spiking blood glucose levels

- Weight gain

- Increased allergies and infections

- Loss of bone density

- Muscle wasting

- Skin thinning

- Inability to build effective proteins and enzymes

- Fluid retention

- Kidney damage

- And, of course, cardio issues. Just think, if there are decreased proteins in the blood, increased fluids in the blood, increased blood sugars, etc. this all depletes the blood vessels and puts more stress on the heart itself.[1]

DHEA (Dhydroepiandrosterone) is a compound produced by the adrenal glands that works in opposition to cortisol. When cortisol goes up, DHEA goes down and visa versa. DHEA attempts to counterbalance the negative immune impact that cortisol has; it tries to protect bone density, and it tries to regulate cholesterols.

Both hyper-adrenal and hypo-adrenal function can have a direct impact on the heart, both directly and indirectly.

For instance, the indirect impact may be the effect the adrenals have on the kidneys, which affect the blood fluids, which in turn affects the heart.

Or the impact may be direct. Epinephrine gets everything flowing at a heightened speed. When the adrenals get going, they also push the heart to pump harder and harder. This can cause symptoms like:

- Heart palpitations
- Panic attacks and/or anxiety attacks
- Shortness of breath

For a more in depth look at the adrenal glands and what they do, please read my book entitled, *Adrenal Fatigue: Why am I so tired all of the time.*

Visit www.choicesunlimited.ca/store

In fact, while adrenaline may be injected in certain cardiac situations, i.e. cardiac arrest (if the heart stops) or extremely low blood pressure, too much adrenaline can cause a heart attack.

So, when it comes to heart health, we have to take stress and the adrenals into consideration as well.

FOURTEEN

Other programs that support a healthy heart

Food is not the only element that can affect the heart. Although we have discussed it only briefly, the impact of psychological stress on the heart cannot be under-estimated.

Programs that can help with stress include:

- Different types of mental focus:
  - Meditation
  - Prayer
  - Contemplation
  - Hypnosis
- Different stress releasers:
  - Pity party time
  - Solution-focused time
  - Singing
  - Breathing exercises
  - Massage

There are other programs that can also help, too. For instance, what about exercise? Do you need to go and get a gym membership and start working out every day? No! In fact, that may even be a detriment. The body, however, is designed for movement.

If there is insufficient movement, we are not helping to:

- Get oxygen into the body
- Get carbon dioxide out of the body
- Get nutrients to the cells
- Move toxins away from the cells
- Move the blood
- Move the lymphatic system
- Move the cerebral spinal fluid
- Keep our bones strong

There are lots of good reasons to move. We don't need to have so much movement we can't absorb anything, like a waterfall. Nor do we want so little movement that we become like a stagnant pond. We want a good healthy moving system that supports all of the above.

I recommend that you start by walking. Walk to the corner and back. When that's comfortable, up the distance to a mile. Gradually increase both your duration and your endurance. Then you can up it again, perhaps adding in a bit of a jog. Make sure you have good runners and are not putting extra stress on the body.

Other good types of exercise include tai chi, yoga, Pilates, stretching, and dance.

What about including biking, skating, or swimming? There are so many ways to get the body moving. Just remember, a healthy body does require movement.

Again work day-by-day and item-by-item and you will find that in no time at all, you have a healthier attitude, body and health. Here's to a healthy heart.

FIFTEEN

Conclusions

Your heart needs you to provide good nutrients to support it so that it can support you. How do you take care of your heart? Here are a few guiding rules:

1. Avoid processed foods.

2. Avoid toxic foods, cleansers, etc.

3. Avoid pharmaceuticals that actually cause more danger than good.

4. Eat healthy whole organic non-GMO foods.

5. Eat healthy fats.

6. Take good supplements.

7. Eat healthy 100% chocolate.

8. Eliminate or find more effective ways of dealing with stress.

There are so many good healthy foods available. Interestingly enough, once you start eating them, you start to crave them. It would appear that as much as unhealthy foods create cravings for the same, healthy foods do likewise. Why? Perhaps part of the equation has to do with the following:

1. When we start to create a healthy profile of gut bacteria, they start to demand the healthy foods.

2. When we start eating healthy, we start to feel better, and a natural association is made within the body and mind for healthier foods.

There might also be another kind of association. When the cells in the body have enough energy and nutrition, they have a stronger capacity to stand up and say: "Hey, I need some healthy nutrients!"

You don't need to change everything as once. That is usually doomed to failure, but if you start by choosing one alternative way of supporting a healthy heart per week it will become easier and easier to accomplish.

Quotes

Chapter 1

[1]Nummenmaa, Lauri, et al. Bodily maps of emotions. Found in: http://www.pnas.org/content/early/2013/12/26/1321 664111

Chapter 2

[1]Random facts and interesting trivia for the curious mind. Found in: http://facts.randomhistory.com/human-heart-facts.html

[2]Heart health: top 8 foods and nutrients. Found in: https://www.cncahealth.com/explore/learn/nutrition-food/heart-health-top-8-foods-and-nutrients

Chapter 3

[1]Meilan, K., et al. Cardiovascular Involvement in General Medical Conditions: Pulmonary diseases and the Heart. Found in: http://circ.ahajournals.org/content/116/25/2992.full

[2]Heart Disease Health Center. Found in: http://www.webmd.com/heart-disease/vascular-disease?page=2

Chapter 4

[1]Mercola, Joseph. Why you shouldn't drink pasteurized milk. Found in: http://www.huffingtonpost.com/dr-mercola/dairy-free-avoid-this-pop_b_558447.html

[2]It seems that most juice in the market is pasteurized. What does this process involve and is pasteurized juice

not a good option when it comes to nutrition? Found in: http://whfoods.org/genpage.php?tname=dailytip&dbid=2 97

[3]Microwaved veg "loses nutrients". Found in: http://news.bbc.co.uk/2/hi/health/3188558.stm

[4]George, DF, et al. Non-thermal effects in the microwave induced unfolding of proteins observed by chaperone binding. Found in: http://www.ncbi.nlm.nih.gov/pubmed/18240290

[5]Microwaving can lower breast milk benefits. Found in: http://www.thefreelibrary.com/Microwaving+can+low er+breast+milk+benefits.-a012100730

[6]Watanabem, F., et al. Effects of Microwave Heating on the Loss of Vitamin B(12) in Foods. Found in: http://www.ncbi.nlm.nih.gov/pubmed/10554220

[7]Pedraza-Chaverri, J., et al. Garlic's ability to prevent in vitro Cu2+ -induced lipoprotein oxidation in human serum is preserved in heated garlic: effect unrelated to Cu2+ -chelation. Found In: http://www.nutritionj.com/content/3/1/10

[8]Hadhazy, Adam. Tip of the Tongue: Human May Have at Least 6 Flavors. Found in: http://www.livescience.com/17684-sixth-basic-taste.html

[9]Roundup Weed Killer. Found in: http://www.motherearthnews.com/nature-and-environment/roundup-weed-killer-zmaz09djzraw.aspx

118

[10]Environmental Toxicity and Body Detoxification. Found In: http://www.hightechhealth.com/enviromental-toxicity

[11]Signs and Symptoms of Pesticide Poisoning. Found in:

http://www.headlice.org/faq/treatments/signs-symptoms.htm#oi

[12]Dioxins and their effects on human health. Found in:

http://www.who.int/mediacentre/factsheets/fs225/en/

[13]PCBs and dioxins in salmon. Found in: http://www.who.int/foodsafety/chem/pcbsalmon/en/

[14]Persistent Organic Pollutants: A Global Issue, A Global Response. Found in:

http://www.epa.gov/oia/toxics/pop.html

[15]Heavy Metals. Found in:

http://www.psr.org/environment-and-health/confronting-toxics/heavy-metals/

[16]Schubert, J., et al. Combined effects in toxicology - a rapid systemic testing procedure: cadmium, mercury, and lead. Found in:

http://www.ncbi.nlm.nih.gov/pubmed/731728

[17]Robin, Suzanne. Healthy Eating. Found in:

http://healthyeating.sfgate.com/foods-containing-mercury-3669.html

[18]Sources of Lead. Found in:
http://www.health.ny.gov/environmental/lead/sources.htm

[19]Lead found in Children's Foods and Baby Foods; Legal Notices Sent to Law Enforcement. Found in: http://www.envirolaw.org/documents/FINALNewsRel ease.pdf

[20]Arsenic in your food: Our findings show a real need for federal standards for this toxin. Found in:

http://consumerreports.org/cro/magazine/2012/11/ar senic-in-your-food/index.htm

[21]Questions and Answers; Arsenic in Rice and Rice Products. Found in:

http://www.fda.gov/Food/FoodborneIllnessContamina nts/Metals/ucm319948.htm

[22]Test Your Food-Safety Smarts. Found in:

http://www.thedailygreen.com/healthy-eating/eat-safe/arsenic-chicken-fda-1310

[23]Aluminum: Public Health Statement. Found in: http://www.atsdr.cdc.gov/toxprofiles/tp22-c1.pdf

[24]How Milk and Dairy Products Will Destroy Your Health and Cause Cancer, Heart Disease, Diabetes, Multiple Sclerosis, Allergies, Osteoporosis, and Infection. Found in:

http://www.all-creatures.org/health/howmilkanddairy.html

[25]EWG's Skin Deep. Found in: http://www.ewg.org/skindeep/site/about.php

[26]The dirt on toxic chemicals in household cleaning products. Found in:

http://www.davidsuzuki.org/issues/health/science/to
xics/the-dirt-on-toxic-chemicals-in-household-cleaning-
products/

[27]Acute Pharma Toxicity. Found in:
http://www.naturalnews.com/027817_acute_pharma_to
xicity_Brittany_Murphy.html

[28]Mercury: The Hidden Trigger to Alzheimer's and
Parkinson's that 75% of People Carry. Found in:
http://articles.mercola.com/sites/articles/archive/2012
/04/07/dangers-of-mercury-contamination.aspx

[29]Wells, S.D. Vaccine Ingredients. Found in:
http://www.naturalnews.com/035431_vaccine_ingredie
nts_side_effects_MSG.html

[30]Vollmer, Sabine. 10 Americans: Industrial toxins found
in umbilical cord blood. Found in:

http://scienceinthetriangle.org/2010/09/10-americans-
industrial-toxins-found-in-umbilical-cord-blood/

[31]Heavy Metal Poisoning Symptoms. Found in:
http://www.evenbetterhealth.com/heavy-metal-
poisoning-symptoms.asp

[32]Warfarin Oral Precautions and Side Effects. Found in:

http://www.healthcentral.com/heart-
disease/r/medications/warfarin-oral-3949/side-
effects?ic=2601

[33]www.HealthCentral.com

[34]Feenstra, Johannes, et al. Drug-induced heart failure.
Found in:

http://content.onlinejacc.org/article.aspx?articleid=1125697

Chapter 5

[1]Ravnskov, Uffe. The Cholesterol Myths : Exposing the Fallacy that Saturated Fat and Cholesterol Cause Heart Disease. 2000, New Trends Publishing, Incorporated. ISBN 0-9670897-0-0.

[2]Lugavere, Max. Your "Healthy" diet could be quietly killing your brain. Found in: http://www.psychologytoday.com/blog/the-optimalist/201310/your-healthy-diet-could-be-quietly-killing-your-brain

[3]Seven Countries Study. Found in: http://en.wikipedia.org/wiki/Seven_Countries_Study

[4]Seven Countries Study. Found in: http://en.wikipedia.org/wiki/Seven_Countries_Study

[5,6,7]The Truth About Ancel Keys: We've all got it Wrong. Found in: http://rawfoodsos.com/2011/12/22/the-truth-about-ancel-keys-weve-all-got-it-wrong/

[8]Keys, Ancel. Human Atherosclerosis and the Diet. Found in: http://circ.ahajournals.org/content/5/1/115.full.pdf

[9]Keys, Ancel. The Relationship of the diet to the development of atherosclerosis. Found in: http://books.google.ca/books?id=c0IrAAAAYAAJa ndpg=PA181andlpg=PA181anddq=keys+anderson+1955 +%22The+relationship+of+the+diet+to+the+developmen t+of+atherosclerosis%22andsource=blandots=9g_j2W-CK4andsig=n3u4urFGrkMTAq4I2UoiiFNAEiUandhl=en

andei=GMvES6n6KZGusgPesezCDgandsa=Xandoi=boo
k_resultandct=resultandredir_esc=y#v=snippetandq=all
%20natural%20diets%20has%20noandf=false

[9]Tatami, R., et al. Intermediate-density lipoprotein and cholesterol-rich very low density lipoprotein in angiographically determined coronary artery disease. Found in:
http://www.ncbi.nlm.nih.gov/pubmed/7296792

[10]Mercola, Joseph. The Cholesterol Myths that May be Harming Your Health. Found in:

http://mercola.ebeaver.org/2011/10/22/the_cholesterol
_myths_that_may_be_harming_your_health/

Chapter 7

[1] Dean, Ward MD., Krebs' Cycle Intermediates: Maximizing Your Body's Performance. Found in:
http://nutritionreview.org/2013/04/krebs-cycle-intermediates/

[2] Fatigue and Nutritional Deficiencies: A Look at the citric Acid Cycle. Found in:
http://spinalalignment.com/articles/nutritional-articles/fatigue-and-nutritional-deficiencies/

[3] Gornik, Heather L., Mark A. Creager. Arginine and Endothelial and Vascular Health. Journal of Nutrition American Society for Nutritional Sciences (2004) Heather L. Gornik and Mark A. Creager. Found in:
jn.nutrition.org/content/134/10/2880S.abstract

[4] What are the benefits of garlic? Found in:
http://www.medicalnewstoday.com/articles/265853.ph
p

Chapter 8

[1]"Citric acid cycle with aconitate 2" by Narayanese, WikiUserPedia, YassineMrabet, TotoBaggins - http://biocyc.org/META/NEW-IMAGE?type=PATHWAY&object=TCA. Image adapted from :Image:Citric acid cycle noi.svg | (uploaded to Commons by wadester16). Licensed under Creative Commons Attribution-Share Alike 3.0 via Wikimedia Commons - http://commons.wikimedia.org/wiki/File:Citric_acid_cycle_with_aconitate_2.svg#mediaviewer/File:Citric_acid_cycle_with_aconitate_2.svg

[2,3]Coenzyme Q10. Found in: http://en.wikipedia.org/wiki/Coq10

[4]This Form of CoQ10 Found Far Superior to One Typically Being Sold. Found in: http://articles.mercola.com/sites/articles/archive/2011/06/29/this-form-of-co-q-10-found-far-superior-to-one-typically-being-sold.aspx

[5]Dixon, Brian, et al. Bioavailability of Ubiquinone versus Ubiquinol. Found in: http://www.usana.com/media/File/dotCom/company/science/crb/UbiquinoneVersusUbiquinol.pdf

[6]Sinatra, Stephen. Choosing a CoQ10 Supplement: Ubiquinol or Ubiquinone? Found in: http://www.drsinatra.com/choosing-a-coq10-supplement-ubiquinol-or-ubiquinone/

[7]Drugs that Deplete: Coenzyme Q10. Found in: https://umm.edu/health/medical/altmed/supplement-depletion-links/drugs-that-deplete-coenzyme-q10

Chapter 9

[1]Mercola, Joseph. My One Hour Vitamin D Lecture to Clear up all Your Confusion on this Vital Nutrient. Found in: http://articles.mercola.com/sites/articles/archive/2008/12/16/my-one-hour-vitamin-d-lecture-to-clear-up-all-your-confusion-on-this-vital-nutrient.aspx

[2]Vitamin D Council: What is Vitamin D? Found in: http://www.vitamindcouncil.org/about-vitamin-d/what-is-vitamin-d/

[3]Meletis, Chris D, ND. Vitamin De: Higher Doses Reduce Risk of Common Health Concerns. Found in: http://www.vrp.com/bone-and-joint/vitamin-d3-higher-doses-reduce-risk-of-common-health-concerns

Chapter 10

[1]Fourchalk, Holly. The Chocolate Controversy: the bad, the mediocre and the Awesome. Found in: www.choicesunlimited.ca/store

Chapter 11

[1]Wong, JM, et al. Gut microbiota, diet, and heart disease. Found in: http://www.ncbi.nlm.nih.gov/pubmed/22468338

[2]Fava, F., et al. The gut microbiota and lipid metabolism: Implications for human health and coronary heart disease. Found in: http://www.ncbi.nlm.nih.gov/pubmed/17073643

[3]Excessive consumption of red meat can change gut microbiota, leading to the appearance of heart disease. Found in:

http://www.gutmicrobiotawatch.org/tag/heart-disease/

Chapter 12

[1]Fallon, Sally, Mary G. Enig. What Causes Heart Disease?
Found
in: http://www.westonaprice.org/cardiovascular-disease/what-causes-heart-disease

[2,3]Huggins, Hal. Root Canal Dangers. Found in:
http://www.westonaprice.org/dentistry/root-canal-dangers

[4]Mercola, Joseph. Mercury: The Hidden Trigger to
Alzheimer's and Parkinson's that 75% of People Carry.
Found in:
http://articles.mercola.com/sites/articles/archive/2012/04/07/dangers-of-mercury-contamination.aspx

[5]What is dental amalgam? What are the dangers of dental
mercury? Found in:
http://www.toxicteeth.org/mercuryfillings.aspx

[6]Hoffman, Jordan. Dental Amalgams and Heavy Metal
Toxicity. Found in:
http://jordanhoffmanacupuncture.com/articles/mercury.htm

[7]Mercola, Joseph. New UN Treaty on Mercury Requires
Countries to Phase Down Dental Amalgam. Found in:
http://articles.mercola.com/sites/articles/archive/2013/02/05/mercury-un-treaty-abolishes-amalgam.aspx

Chapter 13

[1]Northrup, Christiane, MD. Adrenal Exhaustion. Found
in:

http://www.drnorthrup.com/womenshealth/healthcent
er/topic_details.php?topic_id=94

References

Dean, Ward MD., Krebs' Cycle Intermediates: Maximizing Your Body's Performance. Found in: http://nutritionreview.org/2013/04/krebs-cycle-intermediates/

Dixon, Brian, et al. Bioavailability of Ubiquinone versus Ubiquinol. Found in: http://www.usana.com/media/File/dotCom/company/science/crb/UbiquinoneVersusUbiquinol.pdf

Fallon, Sally, Mary G. Enig. What Causes Heart Disease? Found in: http://www.westonaprice.org/cardiovascular-disease/what-causes-heart-disease

Fava, F., et al. The gut microbiota and lipid metabolism: Implications for human health and coronary heart disease. Found in: http://www.ncbi.nlm.nih.gov/pubmed/17073643

Feenstra, Johannes, et al. Drug-induced heart failure. Found in: http://content.onlinejacc.org/article.aspx?articleid=1125697

Fourchalk, Holly. The Chocolate Controversy: the bad, the mediocre and the Awesome. Found in: www.choicesunlimited.ca/store

George, DF, et al. Non-thermal effects in the microwave induced unfolding of proteins observed by chaperone binding. Found in: http://www.ncbi.nlm.nih.gov/pubmed/18240290

Gornik, Heather L., Mark A. Creager. Arginine and Endothelial and Vascular Health. Journal of Nutrition American Society for Nutritional Sciences (2004). Found in: jn.nutrition.org/content/134/10/2880S.abstract

Hadhazy, Adam. Tip of the Tongue: Human May Have at Least 6 Flavors. Found in: http://www.livescience.com/17684-sixth-basic-taste.html

Hoffman, Jordan. Dental Amalgams and Heavy Metal Toxicity. Found in: http://jordanhoffmanacupuncture.com/articles/mercury.htm

Huggins, Hal. Root Canal Dangers. Found in: http://www.westonaprice.org/dentistry/root-canal-dangers

Keys, Ancel. Human Atherosclerosis and the Diet. Found in: http://circ.ahajournals.org/content/5/1/115.full.pdf

Keys, Ancel. The Relationship of the diet to the develop of atherosclerosis. Found in: http://books.google.ca/books?id=c0IrAAAAYAAJa ndpg=PA181andlpg=PA181anddq=keys+anderson+1955 +%22The+relationship+of+the+diet+to+the+developmen t+of+atherosclerosis%22andsource=blandots=9g_j2W-CK4andsig=n3u4urFGrkMTAq4I2UoiiFNAEiUandhl=en andei=GMvES6n6KZGusgPesezCDgandsa=Xandoi=boo k_resultandct=resultandredir_esc=y#v=snippetandq=all %20natural%20diets%20has%20noandf=false

Krucik, Gerge, MD (Colleen Story) types of Heart Disease: All types of heart disease share common traits and have key differences. Learn about the different types, including coronary, ischemic and congenital. Found in: http://www.healthline.com/heart/heart-disease/types#3

Meletis, Chris D, ND. Vitamin De: Higher Doses Reduce Risk of Common Health Concerns. Found in: http://www.vrp.com/bone-and-joint/vitamin-d3-higher-doses-reduce-risk-of-common-health-concerns

Mercola, Joseph. The Cholesterol Myths that May be Harming Your Health. Found in:

http://mercola.ebeaver.org/2011/10/22/the_cholesterol_myths_that_may_be_harming_your_health/

Mercola, Joseph. Why you shouldn't drink pasteurized milk. Found in: http://www.huffingtonpost.com/dr-mercola/dairy-free-avoid-this-pop_b_558447.html

Mercola, Joseph. My One Hour Vitamin D Lecture to Clear up all Your Confusion on this Vital Nutrient. Found in: http://articles.mercola.com/sites/articles/archive/2008/12/16/my-one-hour-vitamin-d-lecture-to-clear-up-all-your-confusion-on-this-vital-nutrient.aspx

Mercola, Joseph. New UN Treaty on Mercury Requires Countries to Phase Down Dental Amalgam. Found in: http://articles.mercola.com/sites/articles/archive/2013/02/05/mercury-un-treaty-abolishes-amalgam.aspx

Mercola, Joseph. Mercury: The Hidden Trigger to Alzheimer's and Parkinson's that 75% of People Carry. Found in:

http://articles.mercola.com/sites/articles/archive/2012/04/07/dangers-of-mercury-contamination.aspx

Northrup, Christiane, MD. Adrenal Exhaustion. Found in: http://www.drnorthrup.com/womenshealth/healthcenter/topic_details.php?topic_id=94

Nummenmaa, Lauri, et al. Bodily maps of emotions. Found in: http://www.pnas.org/content/early/2013/12/26/1321664111

Pedraza-Chaverri, J., et al. Garlic's ability to prevent in vitro Cu2+ -induced lipoprotein oxidation in human serum is preserved in heated garlic: effect unrelated to Cu2+ -chelation. Found In: http://www.nutritionj.com/content/3/1/10

Ravnskov, Uffe. The Cholesterol Myths : Exposing the Fallacy that Saturated Fat and Cholesterol Cause Heart Disease. 2000, New Trends Publishing, Incorporated. ISBN 0-9670897-0-0.

Robin, Suzanne. Healthy Eating. Found in: http://healthyeating.sfgate.com/foods-containing-mercury-3669.html

Schubert, J., et al. Combined effects in toxicology - a rapid systemic testing procedure: cadmium, mercury, and lead. Found in: http://www.ncbi.nlm.nih.gov/pubmed/731728

Seven Countries Study. Found in: http://en.wikipedia.org/wiki/Seven_Countries_Study

Sinatra, Stephen. Choosing a CoQ10 Supplement: Ubiquinol or Ubiquinone? Found in: http://www.drsinatra.com/choosing-a-coq10-supplement-ubiquinol-or-ubiquinone/

Tatami, R., et al. Intermediate-density lipoprotein and cholesterol-rich very low-density lipoprotein in angiographically determined coronary artery disease. Found in: http://www.ncbi.nlm.nih.gov/pubmed/7296792

Vollmer, Sabine. 10 Americans: Industrial toxins found in umbilical cord blood. Found in: http://scienceinthetriangle.org/2010/09/10-americans-industrial-toxins-found-in-umbilical-cord-blood/

Watanabem, F., et al. Effects of Microwave Heating on the Loss of Vitamin B(12) in Foods. Found in: http://www.ncbi.nlm.nih.gov/pubmed/10554220

Wells, S.D. Vaccine Ingredients. Found in: http://www.naturalnews.com/035431_vaccine_ingredients_side_effects_MSG.html

Wong, JM, et al. Gut microbiota, diet, and heart disease. Found in: http://www.ncbi.nlm.nih.gov/pubmed/22468338

Acute Pharma Toxicity. Found in: http://www.naturalnews.com/027817_acute_pharma_toxicity_Brittany_Murphy.html

Aluminum: Public Health Statement. Found in: http://www.atsdr.cdc.gov/toxprofiles/tp22-c1.pdf

Arsenic in your food: Our findings show a real need for federal standards for this toxin. Found in:

http://consumerreports.org/cro/magazine/2012/11/arsenic-in-your-food/index.htm

Coenzyme Q10. Found in:
http://en.wikipedia.org/wiki/Coq10

Dioxins and their effects on human health. Found in:

http://www.who.int/mediacentre/factsheets/fs225/en/

Drugs that Deplete: Coenzyme Q10. Found in:
https://umm.edu/health/medical/altmed/supplement-depletion-links/drugs-that-deplete-coenzyme-q10

Environmental Toxicity and Body Detoxification. Found In: http://www.hightechhealth.com/enviromental-toxicity

EWG's Skin Deep. Found in: http://www.ewg.org/skindeep/site/about.php

Excessive consumption of red meat can change gut microbiota, leading to the appearance of heart disease. Found in:
http://www.gutmicrobiotawatch.org/tag/heart-disease/

Fatigue and Nutritional Deficiencies: A Look at the citric Acid Cycle. Found in:
http://spinalalignment.com/articles/nutritional-articles/fatigue-and-nutritional-deficiencies/

Heart Disease Health Center. Found in:
http://www.webmd.com/heart-disease/vascular-disease?page=2

Heart health: top 8 foods and nutrients. Found in: https://www.cncahealth.com/explore/learn/nutrition-food/heart-health-top-8-foods-and-nutrients

Heavy Metals. Found in: http://www.psr.org/environment-and-health/confronting-toxics/heavy-metals/

Heavy Metal Poisoning Symptoms. Found in: http://www.evenbetterhealth.com/heavy-metal-poisoning-symptoms.asp

How Milk and Dairy Products Will Destroy Your Health and Cause Cancer, Heart Disease, Diabetes, Multiple Sclerosis, Allergies, Osteoporosis, and Infection. Found in: http://www.all-creatures.org/health/howmilkanddairy.html

It seems that most juice in the market is pasteurized. What does this process involve and is pasteurized juice not a good option when it comes to nutrition? Found in: http://whfoods.org/genpage.php?tname=dailytip&dbid=297

Lead found in Children's Foods and Baby Foods; Legal Notices Sent to Law Enforcement. Found in: http://www.envirolaw.org/documents/FINALNewsRelease.pdf

Mercury: The Hidden Trigger to Alzheimer's and Parkinson's that 75% of People Carry. Found in: http://articles.mercola.com/sites/articles/archive/2012/04/07/dangers-of-mercury-contamination.aspx

Microwaved veg "loses nutrients". Found in: http://news.bbc.co.uk/2/hi/health/3188558.stm

Microwaving can lower breast milk benefits. Found in: http://www.thefreelibrary.com/Microwaving+can+lower+breast+milk+benefits.-a012100730

PCBs and dioxins in salmon. Found in: http://www.who.int/foodsafety/chem/pcbsalmon/en/

Persistent Organic Pollutants: A Global Issue, A Global Response. Found in:

http://www.epa.gov/oia/toxics/pop.html

Questions and Answers; Arsenic in Rice and Rice Products. Found in: http://www.fda.gov/Food/FoodborneIllnessContaminants/Metals/ucm319948.htm

Random facts and interesting trivia for the curious mind. Found in: http://facts.randomhistory.com/human-heart-facts.html

Roundup Weed Killer. Found in: http://www.motherearthnews.com/nature-and-environment/roundup-weed-killer-zmaz09djzraw.aspx

Signs and Symptoms of Pesticide Poisoning. Found in: http://www.headlice.org/faq/treatments/signs-symptoms.htm#oiSources of Lead. Found in: http://www.health.ny.gov/environmental/lead/sources.htm

Test Your Food-Safety Smarts. Found in: http://www.thedailygreen.com/healthy-eating/eat-safe/arsenic-chicken-fda-1310

The dirt on toxic chemicals in household cleaning products. Found in: http://www.davidsuzuki.org/issues/health/science/to

xics/the-dirt-on-toxic-chemicals-in-household-cleaning-products/

The Truth About Ancel Keys: We've all got it Wrong. Found in: http://rawfoodsos.com/2011/12/22/the-truth-about-ancel-keys-weve-all-got-it-wrong/

This Form of CoQ10 Found Far Superior to One Typically Being Sold. Found in: http://articles.mercola.com/sites/articles/archive/2011/06/29/this-form-of-co-q-10-found-far-superior-to-one-typically-being-sold.aspx

Vitamin D Council: What is Vitamin D? Found in: http://www.vitamindcouncil.org/about-vitamin-d/what-is-vitamin-d/

Warfarin Oral Precautions and Side Effects. Found in: http://www.healthcentral.com/heart-disease/r/medications/warfarin-oral-3949/side-effects?ic=2601

What is dental amalgam? What are the dangers of dental mercury? Found in: http://www.toxicteeth.org/mercuryfillings.aspx

What are the benefits of garlic? Found in: http://www.medicalnewstoday.com/articles/265853.php

www.HealthCentral.com

www.ingramcontent.com/pod-product-compliance
Lightning Source LLC
Chambersburg PA
CBHW070810290326
41931CB00011BB/2181